Benjamin Black
Bart's & the London

MEDICAL PROTECTION SOCIETY

Supporting your education. Protecting your future.

This Handbook has been supplied to you for FREE by the Medical Protection Society. MPS aims to:

Support your education
We do this by using our buying power to negotiate discounts on books, CD-ROMs and medical journals, this enables us to deliver free and discounted educational materials to you when it matters most.

Protect your future
MPS aims to protect your best interests now and in the future.
As a student this comes in the form of FREE elective protection anywhere in the world.
You will also have access to medico-legal information so that can build on your knowledge of best practice.

To discuss your membership of MPS please call the membership helpline on:
(UK)   0845 718 7187
(Ireland)   1800 509 441

or write to:

Student Membership Services
Medical Protection Society
Granary Wharf House
Leeds
LS11 5PY
www.mps.org.uk/students

MPS Membership number: [   ]

Write your number above in case you ever need to contact us and your contact details below in case you loose this book.

If found please contact/return to:	
Name:	
Medical school:	
Address:	
Telephone:	

Introduction to

CLINICAL EXAMINATION

For Churchill Livingstone:

Commissioning editor: Laurence Hunter
Project development manager: Barbara Simmons
Project manager: Nancy Arnott
Designer: Erik Bigland

INTRODUCTION TO CLINICAL EXAMINATION

Michael J Ford MB ChB (Hons) MD FRCPE

Consultant Physician,
Western General Hospital, Edinburgh;
Clinical Sub-Dean and Part-time Senior Lecturer,
Faculty of Medicine, University of Edinburgh

John F Munro OBE FRCPE FRCP (Glas) FRCP

Retired Consultant Physician,
Eastern General Hospital, Edinburgh;
Honorary Fellow, Faculty of Medicine,
University of Edinburgh

SEVENTH EDITION

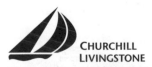

CHURCHILL LIVINGSTONE

EDINBURGH LONDON NEW YORK OXFORD
PHILADELPHIA ST LOUIS SYDNEY TORONTO

CHURCHILL LIVINGSTONE
An imprint of Elsevier Science Limited

First edition 1974
Second edition 1977
Third edition 1983
Fourth edition 1985
Fifth edition 1989
Sixth edition 1993
Seventh edition 2000
  Reprinted 2002

ISBN 0443 063540
International edition 0443 063583
  Reprinted 2002

British Library Cataloguing in Publication Data
A catalogue record for this book is available from the British Library.

Library of Congress Cataloging in Publication Data
A catalog record for this book is available from the Library of
Congress.

Medical knowledge is constantly changing. As new information
becomes available, changes in treatment, procedures, equipment and
the use of drugs become necessary. The author and publisher have,
as far as it is possible, taken care to ensure that the information given
in this text is accurate and up to date. However, readers are strongly
advised to confirm that the information, especially with regard to drug
usage, complies with current legislation and standards of practice.

your source for books,
journals and multimedia
in the health sciences

www.elsevierhealth.com

The
publisher's
policy is to use
**paper manufactured
from sustainable forests**

Printed in China by RDC Group Limited

Preface

The aim of this pocket-book is to provide the medical student with an account of the fundamental methods of clinical examination. It is primarily intended for use at the outset of clinical training, when many feel overwhelmed by detail; senior students should also find the book useful for revision. The text of the seventh edition has been extensively modified. If the primary objective of the book is to describe what to do and how to do it, the secondary objective is to give an indication of when a particular examination is necessary.

The first chapter describes the general principles of history-taking and the last chapter provides a system for integrating the complete physical examination. The other chapters deal with the major systems in turn. Each chapter starts with the cardinal symptoms of disease and the normal physical findings. The method of performing the relevant physical examination is then described in detail using a simple step-by-step procedure. Abnormal findings are described; mention of specific diseases is confined to those which are commonly encountered or which illustrate a specific important point. Most of the methods described can be practised on colleagues so that proficiency can be acquired before the student examines a patient. A simple system of case recording is included at the end of the book.

The ability to undertake a thorough clinical examination is an essential clinical tool. The value of the examination, however, is enhanced by the knowledge of basic science and of disease processes. Such information is available in Macleod's Clinical Examination, 10th edition 2000, edited by Munro and Campbell and published by Churchill Livingstone. The reading of a detailed textbook of this type will be more meaningful after several months of clinical experience. Then the emphasis can be changed from 'how' to 'why' and from the methods of data collection to their interpretation and, with that, the cultivation of critical judgement and independent thought.

Edinburgh, 2000

M.J.F.
J.F.M.

Acknowledgements

The authors wish to thank those past and present authors of the parent textbook, *Macleod's Clinical Examination*, who generously allowed us to adapt their original contributions. The authors are also grateful to many others who have given assistance and constructive criticism. They wish to thank Robert Britton for producing the artwork and Barbara Simmons for all her help in the production of this edition. Finally, they remain indebted to Dr John Macleod and Dr E B French for their invaluable contributions to the earlier editions of this book.

Contents

General principles of history-taking and physical examination 1

Stages of the clinical consultation

- The history
- The physical examination
- The explanation

The **history** is often the most important aspect of the clinical assessment. It is the patient's account of the problem. Properly taken, it should not only describe the current illness but also provide the clinician with information regarding the patient's background and personality. From the history the clinician should know how best to proceed during the physical assessment.

The **physical examination** starts as soon as the clinician meets the patient. Students require to be able to perform a thorough examination, but in practice, the clinician concentrates on those aspects which are relevant.

The **explanation** is from the patient's perspective a critical component of the consultation. The student's role is secondary as the explanation should be given by a clinician with responsibility for the patient's care. To be effective the clinician requires to have gained the patient's confidence by establishing an effective rapport. This skill can be acquired by most students with practice and depends in part upon self-confidence (see Table 1).

Table 1
Aspects of establishing rapport
• Welcome in a warm, friendly manner
• Maintain good eye contact
• Make physical contact as appropriate
• Listen attentively
• Avoid being judgemental

Many junior students feel intimidated. Most patients, however, are keen to put the apprehensive student at ease! If the consultation is considered to be discussion between two experts, the quality of the rapport that is established is likely to be more effective. Students should learn to acquire a professional attitude and, at the same time, be seen to be caring and compassionate. They need to be tolerant at all times, particularly with the elderly and the deaf. They should remember that they are not directly responsible for the patient's medical care and that some individuals may try to obtain from them opinions about diagnosis or treatment. Such enquiries should be referred to the medical staff. Other patients may tell students in confidence about highly personal details. Students should listen to such comments without showing embarrassment and then try to obtain the patient's consent to discuss these with a member of the medical staff as they may be of importance in the patient's management. The student can learn much about the complex interactions between patient and doctor by attempting to analyse unusual feelings aroused by patients and discussing problems of this type with a tutor.

HISTORY

The essential skill of history-taking involves the ability to be flexible while, at the same time, being methodical and systematic in approach. It is important to give the patient undivided attention during the history. Some clinicians dictate a record of the history after it has been obtained; others take detailed notes while the patient is speaking. However, it is best to stop writing if a sensitive subject is being discussed.

There is no correct way to obtain a history. One effective sequence comprises:

- The introduction
- The presenting complaint:
  - Patient's account
  - Supplementary enquiry
- The systemic enquiry
- Drugs and allergies
- Past history
- Family history
- Social and personal history.

Introduction

Students should introduce themselves, giving their name and status and a friendly greeting. They should explain the purpose of their visit, ask for and remember the patient's name and request permission to interview and examine the patient. Some patients may decline because they feel ill, or are tired of being questioned and examined, or are depressed or apprehensive. If difficulties are encountered, the student should consult with the medical or nursing staff.

The presenting complaint

This comprises obtaining the patient's description of the illness and then, as necessary, asking supplementary questions to clarify the story.

The patient's account

It is often valuable to invite the patient to start by briefly mentioning any previous serious illnesses. The patient should then be asked to speak about current problems by an opening remark such as: 'Please tell me about your present trouble' or 'When were you last well?' followed by 'What has happened since?' Students should learn to become good listeners and to avoid the temptation to interrupt the history by asking specific questions which are better asked later in the interview. The patient should be encouraged to continue the story right up to the time of interview. When given the opportunity many patients will provide much information about their illness and themselves. They often need to talk about their troubles, and clinicians who recognise this and are good listeners usually establish good relationships quickly. However, it is necessary to steer the talkative individual from less relevant detail or to help the inarticulate patient by posing simple questions.

Some patients may be unable to give a history because they are too ill, confused or demented. In such circumstances further information should be obtained from a relative or neighbour and the general practitioner. This will also help to establish the history in patients who may be evasive for other reasons, such as alcohol or drug abuse.

The supplementary enquiry

When the patient has completed the account of the current illness, the next step is to clarify the description by specific questioning to obtain a detailed chronological account of the development of the illness from the first symptom to the time of interview. Vague statements such as 'a short while ago' require clarification. It may be necessary to obtain much more detailed information about specific symptoms, e.g. pain (Table 2).

Additional specific questions that may require to be asked will depend upon the nature of the principal complaint. A knowledge of the relevant questions can only be acquired with time. However, as an illustrative example, the specific questions that might be put to a patient presenting with renal colic include the following:

- Recent weight loss
- Recent bone pain (hyperparathyroidism)
- Prolonged bed rest or immobility
- Current drugs and medication, especially vitamin D
- NSAID ingestion, e.g. aspirin ingestion (papillary necrosis)
- Milk – alkali ingestion
- Past history of urinary tract infection

Table 2
Analysis of pain

- Main site
- Radiation
- Character
- Severity
- Duration
- Frequency and periodicity
- Special times of occurrence
- Aggravating factors
- Relieving factors
- Associated phenomena

- Past history of renal colic
- History of diabetes mellitus (papillary necrosis)
- History of chronic alcohol abuse (papillary necrosis)
- Family history of renal stones
- Family or past history of gout.

Questions should be simple and without bias, but the history may be misleading if the patient's interpretations are accepted uncritically; for example, 'flu' or 'rheumatism' may indicate a serious disease. It is important to identify which investigations and treatments have been performed and what the patient has been told about the present illness. History-taking should include details of complaints and events right up to the time of the interview.

Summary points

✦ Let patients tell their own story.
✦ Use open questions at the start.
✦ Use specific (closed) questions later.
✦ Clarify patients' statements and diagnoses.
✦ Steer patients towards the relevant.
✦ Conclude the history with today's events.
✦ Summarise the story.

Systemic enquiry

Significant symptoms may not be mentioned because of embarrassment or because they appear unimportant to the patient. Questions should therefore be asked about principal symptoms concerning the major systems, as described in the various systemic chapters. Lay terms can be used deliberately to broaden the scope of the systemic enquiry, e.g. indigestion; these then may require further clarification.

Drugs and allergies

It is essential to know about the patient's current and previous medication, as any drug may cause ill effects. Some, such as anticoagulants or corticosteroids, are potentially so dangerous that the patient should carry a card giving details of the treatment. If there is doubt about the precise nature of any recent medication, the patient should be asked to produce the pills for identification. Any allergy should be recorded in a conspicuous position in the patient's notes.

Past history

In addition to the initial list of previous illnesses, it may be helpful to know about the outcome of any medical or radiological examination carried out for employment or insurance purposes and to know about the patient's immunisation status, e.g. tetanus, rubella and tuberculosis. Similarly, it is important to ask about any travel or residence abroad. When infection is suspected and the cause is not immediately obvious, it is vital to ask 'Have you ever been abroad?'

Family history

The frequency of inherited and environmental factors in the aetiology of disease makes it essential to know about the age and health, or cause of death, of the patient's parents, spouse, siblings and other close relatives. A method of recording the family history is shown in Figure 1 and illustrated by an inherited disorder.

Social and personal history

An individual's health and well-being are affected by occupational, social and personal factors. Knowledge of the individual's background may be important in making the diagnosis and necessary for planning the management. For example, an elderly patient living alone will almost certainly require different support from one living with a devoted daughter. A social history is especially important when assessing the elderly, confused and those with any chronic disability, particularly if they live alone. Activities of daily living (ADL) include bathing, dressing, toileting and shopping.

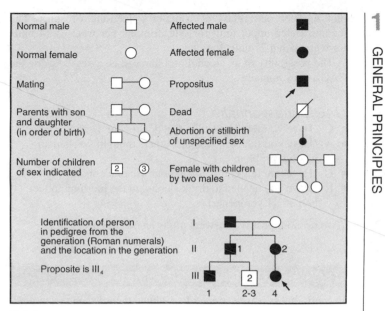

Fig. 1
Note the symbols used in pedigree charts. It may be useful to draw the family tree beginning with the affected person first found to have the trait (propositus if male, proposita if female). Thereafter, all the relevant information regarding siblings and all maternal and paternal relatives should be included.

The patient's ability to cope can be best assessed by asking relevant questions such as:

- Can you use the bath or shower without assistance?
- Can you manage to use the toilet without assistance?
- How long does it take you to get dressed and can you dress without help?
- How far can you walk on level ground without stopping?
- Do you have difficulty opening tins, bottles or cartons?

How patients live, think and behave will also influence how they cope with illness. It is important to obtain details of the patient's lifestyle and personal relationships. Enquiry should therefore be made about employment status, housing, personal and sexual relationships (or lack of them), leisure interests, physical exercise and the use of recreational drugs, including tobacco and alcohol. Alcohol intake can be assessed in terms of units consumed per week; 1 unit comprises 10 g of alcohol equivalent to half of pint of beer or a glass of wine or a measure of spirit. The recommended upper limit for safe drinking per week is 14 units for women and 21 units for men.

The possibility of an alcohol problem can be assessed using the CAGE questionnaire.

CAGE questionnaire
- **C** 'Have you felt the need to **C**ut down your alcohol intake?'
- **A** 'Have you felt **A**nnoyed that others thought you had an alcohol problem?'
- **G** 'Have you felt **G**uilty about your use of alcohol?'
- **E** 'Have you needed to drink alcohol in the morning to feel better?' (**E**ye-opener).

(Two or more positive answers imply an alcohol problem.)

PSYCHOLOGICAL ASSESSMENT

In every illness it is necessary to evaluate the relevant psychological factors. The account of the history and the manner in which it is given usually reveal much about the patient's personality and emotional state. A patient who becomes upset at any stage of the proceedings should be encouraged to talk, as this may reveal a problem such as an unsatisfactory personal relationship or a bereavement. If it becomes apparent that the patient has a psychological difficulty, a more detailed psychological assessment is indicated.

Basic elements of psychological assessment
- Psychological history
- Examination of the mental state
- Examination of intellectual function (p. 66)
- Evaluation of the personality

Psychological history

The history should be taken in private and comfort. The clinician should encourage the patient to speak about personal experiences, and act as a guide rather than an interrogator. Sensitive subjects, such as sex or bereavement, should be discussed frankly and directly without embarrassment. Indeed, enquiry may be welcomed by a depressed patient as a much needed opportunity to disclose suicidal thoughts. The clinician collates information as it emerge about the relationships the patient has with each parent and sibling, the adaptation made to schooling and to puberty, adolescent friendships, the development of independence, employment, courtship and marriage, and about attitudes towards spouse and children. Gaps can be filled by specific enquiry towards the end of the interview.

Examination of the mental state

General appearance and behaviour
○ Assess the patient's expressions, dress and reactions.

Thought processes
○ Assess the patient's speech and expression of concepts.
○ Record a sample of the patient's talk and speech content.

Mood (affect)
○ Assess the patient's mood and state of mind.
- 'How have you been feeling in your spirits lately?'
- 'Have you felt worried, tense or irritable recently?'
- 'Do you have any difficulties in sleeping?'
- 'Do you feel brighter in the mornings or evenings'
- 'Has life seemed less worthwhile lately?'
- 'Have you had thoughts of suicide recently?'

Delusions and hallucinations
○ Look for evidence of delusions (false beliefs).
○ Ask about experiences of visual or auditory hallucinations.
○ 'Have you seen or heard things that others have been unaware of?'

EVALUATION OF THE PERSONALITY

The patient's general appearance, dress, behaviour, mannerisms and expressions helps in the assessment of the patient's personality and may indicate features suggesting dependent, obsessive or schizoid personalities.

Summary points

✦ A good history takes time and patience.
✦ Listening is more important than speaking.

+ Many patients are at least as frightened as the student.
+ Understanding lessens fear for both patient and student.
+ The method of taking the history influences what the patient says.
+ The history is usually more important than the physical examination in making the diagnosis.
+ Explanation is an intrinsic part of the consultation. Good rapport is a prerequisite for effective communication.

RELATING THE PHYSICAL EXAMINATION TO THE HISTORY

A detailed history is usually more helpful in making the correct diagnosis than is the physical examination. The history should also direct the clinician to making the appropriate examination.

GENERAL PRINCIPLES OF THE PHYSICAL EXAMINATION

○ Privacy and warmth are essential; in a hospital ward or out-patient department, draw the screens round the bed or couch before the examination.

○ Illumination should be good; exposure of the area to be examined should be adequate but not to an extent that might unnecessarily embarrass or chill the patient.

○ Ensure that both patient and the examiner are warm; apart from the discomfort, shivering causes muscle sounds which interfere with auscultation, while abdominal palpation with cold hands will cause the muscles to contract during the examination.

○ Much of the clinical examination is best conducted from the patient's right side if the clinician is right-handed (and from the patient's left side if left-handed).

○ Examine the patient as thoroughly as possible without causing exhaustion; the risk of this occurring is greatest in the sick, frail or elderly. Sometimes, it is best to complete the examination in several visits.

○ Handle any painful area as gently as possible.

○ Breathless patients should be examined semirecumbent as they will be more breathless lying flat.

○ Young female patients require special consideration by male students. Ask the medical or nursing staff for advice about chaperoning.

○ Record the examination findings systematically (p. 128). Use diagrams to define the site and extent of physical findings such as swellings or the effects of trauma (p. 51).

○ Identify the patient's problems and then decide on a management plan, further investigations and an outline of the treatment.

The cardiovascular system 2

HISTORY

Cardinal symptoms of heart disease

- Chest pain
- Breathlessness
- Oedema
- Palpitation

○ **Chest pain** due to myocardial ischaemia (*angina pectoris*) is characteristically brought on by an increase in cardiac work as induced by exercise or intense emotion. It is relieved by rest within a few minutes. In contrast, the pain of myocardial infarction may commence when the patient is at rest and usually lasts for 20 minutes or longer. Cardiac pain should be analysed as outlined on page 5. The pain is usually described as a 'tightness' or 'heaviness', sometimes as 'indigestion' or even 'breathlessness'. The main site is usually retrosternal. Radiation commonly occurs to the left shoulder and arm, but the pain may be felt exclusively in either or both arms, the neck, jaws, back and epigastrium. The pain of myocardial infarction may be accompanied by breathlessness, nausea, sweating and a sensation of impending doom (*angor animi*).

○ **Breathlessness** occurring on exertion and relieved by rest is usually the earliest symptom of left heart failure. It is due to decreased lung compliance caused initially by pulmonary venous congestion. Sometimes the patient may be wakened from sleep by breathlessness due to acute pulmonary oedema and be forced to sit up to obtain relief (*paroxysmal nocturnal dyspnoea*); cough and watery, frothy and sometimes blood-stained sputum are frequent accompanying features. Breathlessness associated with lying flat is known as *orthopnoea*. Nocturnal dyspnoea and orthopnoea may also occur in obstructive airways disease, including asthma.

○ **Oedema** of cardiac origin is due to the hydrostatic effects of cardiac failure and changes in renal function causing salt and water retention. It is most marked in dependent areas and is usually first noticed at the ankles.

○ **Palpitation** is an awareness of the heart beat. This can be caused by fright, anxiety, ectopic beats or arrhythmias. The patient should be asked to illustrate the frequency and rhythm by tapping a finger on the chest.

○ **Syncope** is sudden transient loss of consciousness; presyncope is the sensation of faintness without loss of consciousness. Both may be cardiac in origin; for example, secondary to a cardiac arrhythmia.

None of these symptoms is specific to heart disease; for example, chest pain may be oesophageal and breathlessness respiratory in origin. Conversely, patients with heart disease may have non-specific symptoms or be asymptomatic.

Symptoms of arterial disease

Acute and chronic ischaemia due to arterial insufficiency leads to symptoms which are determined by the anatomical site, commonly the heart, brain and lower limbs. Arterial insufficiency is much more common in the legs than in the arms. Acute ischaemia may be thrombotic or embolic in origin; chronic ischaemia is usually caused by atheroma.

Ischaemic syndromes
- The heart: *acute* – myocardial infarction; or *chronic* – angina pectoris.
- The brain: *acute* – cerebral infarction, i.e. stroke resulting in neurological deficits such as hemiplegia; or *chronic* – cerebrovascular (multi-infarct) dementia.
- The legs: *acute* – arterial embolism; or chronic – intermittent claudication, i.e. pain in the calf muscles on walking relieved by rest.

Symptoms of venous disease

Thrombosis of a major vein in the leg may cause local pain, tenderness, warmth and swelling. However, major venous thrombosis may remain undetected unless a pulmonary embolus develops resulting in symptoms such as collapse, breathlessness, pleural pain or haemoptysis. The clinical manifestations of venous obstruction depend on its site and extent, together with the adequacy of collateral vessels. Varicose veins are usually obvious and may be cosmetically distressing but otherwise asymptomatic. They are typically confined to the long saphenous system.

PHYSICAL EXAMINATION

This is usually begun with a general inspection of the patient, particular attention being paid to breathlessness and cyanosis. Thereafter, the examination comprises the radial and other arterial pulses and the jugular venous pulse. The heart is examined by inspection, palpation and auscultation. Signs of cardiac failure in other systems are sought in the lungs, liver, trunk and legs. Inspection of the fundus oculi for arterial changes, haemorrhages, exudates and papilloedema is particularly relevant in arterial hypertension. The blood pressure should be recorded, in both the supine and erect positions.

RADIAL PULSE

The radial pulse is examined at the wrist for rate, rhythm and vessel wall. An assessment of volume and wave form is best made by examining a major vessel, such as the carotid artery in the neck.

○ **Rate.** The average of 72 beats per minute in adults rises in response to exercise, anxiety, fever or hyperthyroidism. Resting pulse rates of 40 or less may be due to heart block, and of more than 120 may be due to ectopic foci becoming 'pacemakers' as in paroxysmal tachycardia.

○ **Rhythm.** This is normally regular, though, especially in the young, the rate may quicken on inspiration (*sinus arrhythmia*). Irregular rhythm is most commonly due to frequent ectopic beats or atrial fibrillation.

○ **Form of the pulse wave.** The wave may rise more suddenly than normal when diastolic pressure is low but systolic pressure well maintained. The resultant slapping sensation is increased by raising the arm (and decreased by lowering it) owing to the hydrostatic effect on blood pressure. This '*collapsing pulse*' is most striking in severe aortic incompetence. By contrast, a prolonged wave of low amplitude is characteristic of stenosis of the aortic valve.

○ **Volume.** Providing that the form of the pulse wave and the calibre and elasticity of the artery are normal, the size of the wave is proportional to left ventricular stroke volume. In severe asthma and cardiac tamponade, pulse volume may be dramatically reduced during inspiration owing to fall in venous return, a phenomenon known as '*pulsus paradoxus*'.

○ **Vessel wall.** Hardening and tortuosity are usually due to Monckeberg's medial sclerosis, a nonocclusive arterial disease of little importance, commonly found in the elderly.

Examination sequence

❑ Place 2–3 fingers over the artery.

- Assess the rate and rhythm by counting for at least 30 seconds.

- Obliterate the radial pulse with firm pressure before assessing the state of the vessel wall with the middle finger.

PERIPHERAL VASCULAR SYSTEM

Inspection, palpation and auscultation are the methods employed.

Examination sequence

- Compare the two limbs for pallor, cyanosis and evidence of nutritional changes.

- Compare the temperature of the two limbs using the back of the hand, moving from proximal to distal.

- Check the time taken for capillary refilling after blanching the skin over the foot and the toes.

- Detect the dorsalis pedis pulse using fingertips placed immediately lateral to the extensor hallucis longus tendon and proximal to the first metatarsal space.

- Find the posterior tibial pulse behind the medial malleolus.

- To locate the popliteal pulse, place both thumbs on the patella and curl the fingers of both hands firmly into the popliteal fossa with the knee slightly flexed.

- Palpate the femoral pulse at the mid-inguinal point.

- Palpate the main pulses in the upper limbs and neck.

- Assess the volume and waveform using the carotid, brachial or femoral artery.

- Place the stethoscope lightly on the skin and auscultate over the major vessels (carotid, subclavian, abdominal aorta, renal and femoral arteries).

- 'Walk' the stethoscope along the line of the vessels.
○ **An arterial bruit** indicates turbulence of flow. It may be audible over, and distal to, the site of stenosis of a major artery, such as the abdominal aorta, and the internal carotid, subclavian, femoral or renal arteries (Fig. 2). The possibility of a renal bruit should be sought in any patient presenting with hypertension. A

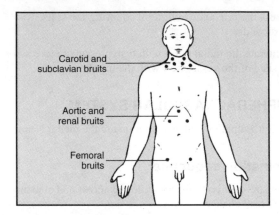

Fig. 2
Sites to listen for major arterial bruits.

systolic bruit over the abdominal aorta may be present in a healthy subject.

○ **Arterial insufficiency** is best detected by looking for any differences in the peripheral pulses (Fig. 3) or in the temperature and nutritional status of the two limbs. Signs of arterial insufficiency are most marked at the periphery of a limb. Signs of acute arterial insufficiency include rest pain, weakness, sensory impairment, coldness and pallor or cyanosis. Features of chronic arterial insufficiency include exercise-induced pain (intermittent claudication, see p. 15) and nutritional changes, e.g. failure of nail growth, loss of hairs and atrophy of subcutaneous tissue of the digits.

In acute arterial insufficiency, the limb feels cold; in contrast, in chronic arterial insufficiency a collateral circulation develops, and the limb, though still inadequately supplied with blood at the core, may feel warmer because of the dilated arteries in the skin. When the foot pulses are present it is not necessary to palpate more proximal pulses. However, students should take every opportunity of improving their technique for palpating the popliteal pulse. The normal popliteal pulse feels forcible and lies in or near the midline of the popliteal fossa.

Examination sequence

Proximal deep vein thrombosis

❏ Compare the colour of both legs and look for cyanosis of the skin and toenails.

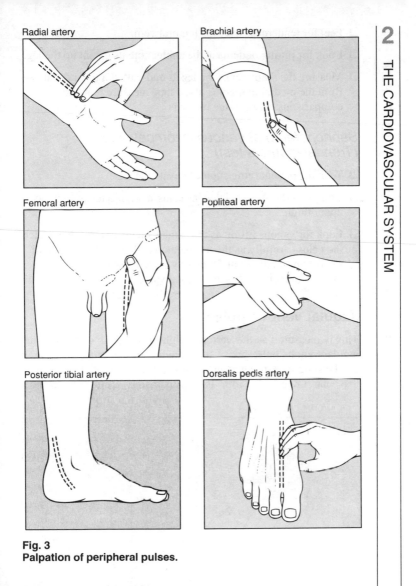

Radial artery

Brachial artery

Femoral artery

Popliteal artery

Posterior tibial artery

Dorsalis pedis artery

**Fig. 3
Palpation of peripheral pulses.**

❑ Look for venous distension and check to see if the veins empty promptly on elevation.

❑ Gently palpate the calf for evidence of heat and tenderness but avoid unnecessary handling.

19

❑ Feel for tenderness over the femoral vein.

❑ Look for pitting oedema at the ankle; note its extent up the leg.

❑ Measure the diameter of the leg at mid-calf at a fixed distance from the medial malleolus; use a tape measure to make comparisons between the two legs.

Saphenofemoral venous incompetence (Trendelenburg's test)

❑ With the patient lying supine, elevate the leg.

❑ Compress the superficial veins using a tourniquet around the upper thigh.

❑ Look for venous filling as the patient stands upright then watch the veins carefully as the tourniquet is released. Veins that fill slowly on standing but fill rapidly on releasing the tourniquet have incompetent saphenofemoral valves.

Jugular venous pulse

This is measured as the vertical height of the peak of the internal jugular venous pulse above the manubriosternal angle (Fig. 4). It can be roughly estimated in centimetres of blood if it is assumed that one finger's breadth is approximately 2 cm. The normal

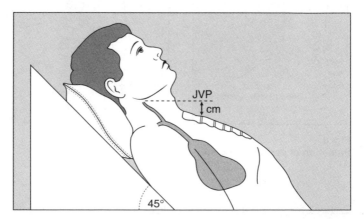

Fig. 4
Estimation of the jugular venous pressure. The observer is looking for the uppermost point of distension of the right internal jugular vein deep to the sternomastoid muscle.

venous pressure is less than 3 cm and falls during inspiration. Thus, in a healthy person reclining at 45 degrees, the jugular venous pulse (JVP) should not be seen above the level of the clavicle. Persistent elevation of the jugular venous pressure is the earliest and most reliable sign of right ventricular failure. Normally the 'a' and 'v' waves are visible if the patient lies down sufficiently to bring the venous pulse into view (Fig. 5).

Examination sequence

❏ Position the patient reclining at 45 degrees to the horizontal, and with the head turned to the left.

❏ Inspect the neck carefully for any pulsation deep to the sternomastoid; distinguish the carotid artery pulse from internal jugular venous pulsation; the former is readily palpable and does not alter with respiration, patient position or compression of the abdomen.

❏ Compress the abdomen to identify the internal jugular vein by the visible rise in venous pulsation (*'hepatojugular reflux'*). If doubt remains, compress the internal jugular vein to distinguish between venous and arterial pulsation.

❏ If necessary, reposition the patient to assess the waveform and identify the components of the JVP.

◯ **The a wave** is due to atrial systole. It is exaggerated when the right atrium contracts against increased resistance, as in right ventricular hypertrophy. The a waves disappear in the absence of

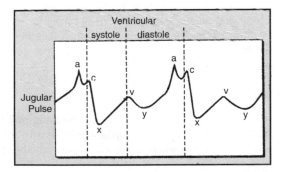

Fig. 5
Form of the venous pulse wave. a = atrial systole; c = onset of ventricular systole; v = peak pressure in right atrium at opening of tricuspid valve; a – x = x descent, due to atrial relaxation; v – y = y descent at commencement of ventricular filling.

atrial contraction, e.g. atrial fibrillation, and are particularly prominent when atrial contraction occurs while the tricuspid valve is closed, '*cannon waves*', as in atrioventricular dissociation.

○ **The c wave** is not clinically detectable and is due to the impulse transmitted from the adjacent carotid artery.

○ **The v wave** is due to venous filling during ventricular systole, and peaks immediately before the opening of the tricuspid valve. When there is tricuspid regurgitation, a positive, systolic '*v wave*' due to the regurgitation of blood into the atrium replaces the usual dip in pressure in early systole.

EXAMINATION OF THE HEART

Inspection

The apex beat may be visible on inspection and is normally in the fifth intercostal space and medial to the midclavicular line.

Examination sequence

❑ Position the patient semirecumbent and relaxed, with the head comfortably supported.

❑ Note any asymmetry of the chest wall which may have displaced the heart.

❑ Inspect the precordium for the apical impulse and other pulsations.

Other pulsations sometimes visible include a left parasternal movement due to right ventricular hypertrophy, and a pulsation in the second left intercostal space arising from an enlarged pulmonary artery. Retraction or pulsation is often seen high in the epigastrium owing to contraction of the heart or expansion of the abdominal aorta, respectively.

Palpation

The precordium is palpated for normal and abnormal pulsations and for thrills. The apex beat is the furthest point downwards and outwards on the chest wall where the apical impulse can be found.

Examination sequence

❑ To examine the apex beat, first place the right hand on the left chest wall and assess its character. Then localise the impulse with a finger-tip.

❑ Identify the position of the apex beat by 'counting down' from the second intercostal space, below the manubriosternal junction and laterally in relation to the midclavicular line. If displaced laterally, check the position of the trachea (p. 37).

❑ Place the thenar eminence of the right hand on the right and left side of the sternum to identify and localise parasternal heaves.

❑ Thrills are best detected by palpating the valve areas with the patient in the optimum position to hear the associated murmur (see below).

The apex beat is commonly impalpable in patients with a thick chest wall or emphysema. It may be displaced by deformity of the chest wall or spine, by diseases of the lungs or pleura, or by cardiac enlargement. The apical impulse is abnormally forceful in left ventricular hypertrophy and is described as '*heaving*' or '*thrusting*' in character, whereas a '*tapping*' sensation is felt in mitral stenosis due to a loud first heart sound on closure of the mitral valve. Palpation of the rest of the precordium may reveal a left parasternal heave due to right ventricular hypertrophy or some other abnormal movement. A murmur may be so loud as to be palpable as a '*thrill*' (i.e. a vibrating sensation).

Auscultation

The earpieces of the stethoscope should fit comfortably and the spring should be strong enough to hold them firmly in place. The tubing should be about 25 cm in length and thick enough to reduce external noise. The diaphragm produces greater sound amplification especially of higher-pitched sounds; the bell is better for the detection of lower-pitched sounds and should be applied lightly on the skin in contrast to the diaphragm which should be pressed firmly against the skin. With modern stethoscopes designed for optimal acoustics, the diaphragm can be used for most purposes; indeed, some stethoscopes no longer have a bell. Many clinicians listen first to the apex, but others prefer to start in the second left intercostal space where both components of the normal second heart sound are best heard (Fig. 6). This provides a reliable point of orientation in the cardiac cycle.

Examination sequence

❑ Auscultate over all the precordium and the great vessels.

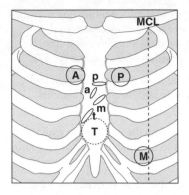

**Fig. 6
Position of the heart valves
and auscultatory areas.
The latter are arbitrary sites
in the neighbourhood of
which murmurs from the
relevant valves are usually
but not always preferentially
heard. MCL = mid-clavicular
line**

❑ Identify the first and second heart sounds; note their character, intensity and any splitting.

❑ Now auscultate the interval between the heart sounds for added sounds and murmurs.

❑ Roll the patient into the semilateral position when listening at the apex. Use the bell pressed lightly on the skin to detect mitral diastolic murmurs which are low-pitched.

❑ Sit the patient forward with the breath held in expiration while auscultating at the left sternal edge. Use the diaphragm pressed firmly against the skin to detect high-pitched aortic diastolic murmurs.

❑ Note the site, timing, character, pitch, radiation and intensity of any murmur.

Heart sounds

The relationship of the heart sounds and added sounds to the electrocardiograph is shown in Figure 7.

○ **The first heart sound** (S1) is best heard at the apex and is mainly due to closure of the mitral valve, the tricuspid component being minor. The intensity is reduced in mitral regurgitation and increased in the presence of mitral stenosis, when its quality is more abrupt in keeping with the 'tapping' apex beat. The first heart sound varies in intensity in the presence of an irregular rhythm or complete heart block.

○ **The second heart sound** (S2) is best heard at the left sternal edge in the second intercostal space. It is caused by closure of the aortic and pulmonary valves. During inspiration, closure of the pulmonary valve is delayed, producing the normal physiological

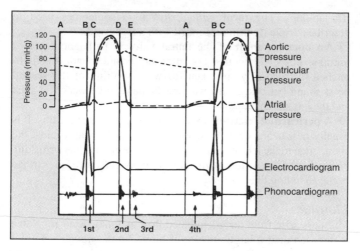

Fig. 7
The relationship between heart sounds, the electrocardiogram and the cardiac cycle in the left side of the heart. A = initiation of atrial contraction; B = closure of mitral valve; C = opening of aortic valve; D = closure of aortic valve; E = opening of mitral valve; B–D = clinical systole; D–B = clinical diastole, subdivided into early diastole (D–E), mid-diastole (E–A) and presystole (A–B).

splitting. Any process which further delays closure will accentuate this splitting, e.g. pulmonary hypertension, right bundle branch block or left-to-right intracardiac shunts. Reversed splitting, heard on expiration, occurs when closure of the aortic valve is delayed, as in left bundle branch block.

Added sounds
○ **The third heart sound** (S3) imparts a typical cadence to the heart sounds 'Lup-dup-dum' – *S1 – S2 – S3*. It is commonly heard at the apex in healthy children and young adults, occurs during early ventricular filling and is low-pitched and best heard using the bell of the stethoscope. When audible in older people it is usually indicative of cardiac failure. It is also a common feature of mitral incompetence.
○ **The fourth heart sound** (S4) is coincident with atrial contraction and thus precedes the first heart sound. It is low-pitched and associated with atrial hypertrophy. It may occur in systemic hypertension and imparts a typical cadence to the heart sounds

'Da-lup-dup'. The term *gallop rhythm* is sometimes used to describe a triple rhythm associated with a tachycardia.

○ **An opening snap** of the mitral valve is pathognomonic of mitral stenosis and occurs soon after the second sound. It is high-pitched, occasionally mistaken for wide splitting of the second heart sound but best heard with the diaphragm between the apex and the left sternal edge.

○ **A pericardial friction rub** is characteristic of pericarditis. It is usually best heard with the diaphragm pressed firmly against the chest, often to the left of the lower end of the sternum. It is a creaking or rustling noise often with three components in each cardiac cycle, sounding like '*chi-te-chi*'.

Murmurs

Murmurs arise from turbulent blood flow and may occur if a valve is diseased or if a large amount of blood flows through a normal valve.

○ **Site.** The area over which a murmur is best heard depends upon the valve of origin or cardiac defect and the directions of the blood flow (Fig. 6). Mitral murmurs are best heard at the apex and aortic systolic murmurs are often maximal in the second intercostal space to the right of the sternal edge (Fig. 8).

○ **Radiation** occurs along the line of blood flow. It follows that an aortic mid-systolic (ejection) murmur radiates into the neck, and an aortic diastolic (regurgitant) murmur radiates down the left sternal edge (Fig. 8).

○ **Pitch** may be characteristic. As a general principle, the greater the pressure gradient, the higher the pitch. The murmur of mitral stenosis is low-pitched, whereas that of aortic regurgitation (incompetence) is high-pitched.

○ **Timing.** Murmurs are timed in relation to the first and second heart sounds. The heart sounds are usually readily identified at the base of the heart, where the second heart sound is usually the louder. The first heart sound can also be identified by its coincidence with the apical impulse; if this is impalpable, then the carotid pulse may be used. The radial pulse is unsuitable as it is delayed by about 0.15 s. Murmurs are usually systolic or diastolic (Fig. 9). Rarely, they may be both, e.g. the continuous murmur of a persistent ductus arteriosus.

○ **Systole** is defined clinically as the time between the first and second heart sounds during which the mitral and tricuspid valves are closed. A systolic murmur arising at the aortic valve is mid-systolic, as flow does not start until ventricular pressure reaches aortic diastolic pressure; it then increases and finally tapers off

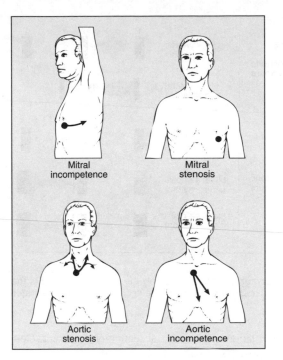

Fig. 8
Murmurs: areas of maximum intensity and selective radiation.

before the aortic valve closes to cause a 'diamond-shaped' ejection systolic murmur. The mitral regurgitant murmur starts with the first heart sound and continues throughout systole, producing a pansystolic murmur that continues beyond and may partially obscure the second heart sound.

○ **Diastole** is defined clinically as the time between the second and the first heart sounds and can be divided into three phases. Early diastole extends from the closing of the aortic and pulmonary valves to the opening of the mitral and tricuspid valves. In mid-diastole, passive filling of the ventricles occurs. Presystole comprises atrial systole up to the closing of the mitral and tricuspid valves. It follows that aortic regurgitant murmurs commence in early diastole and extend into mid-diastole. The murmur of mitral stenosis commences in mid-diastole and is accentuated by atrial contraction during presystole. Sometimes, only the presystolic component can be heard in mitral stenosis, but if there is

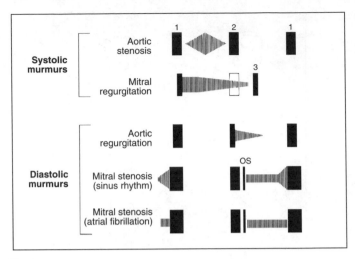

Fig. 9
Heart murmurs. For simplicity only the mitral component of the first
sound and aortic component of the second sound are illustrated.

atrial fibrillation, presystolic accentuation is absent. Comparable
murmurs arise less commonly in the right side of the heart.
○ **Intensity.** The intensity of murmurs may be an index of their
clinical significance. Murmurs may change in intensity. For example,
with increasing degrees of aortic incompetence, the murmur will
become louder. However, murmurs may also diminish in intensity
when the volume of blood flowing through the valve is reduced. A
change in grade is usually clinically significant.

Grades of murmur intensity:
Grade 1: just audible by an expert in optimal conditions
Grade 2: quiet; just audible by a non-expert in optimal conditions
Grade 3: moderately loud
Grade 4: loud and accompanied by a palpable thrill
Grade 5: very loud
Grade 6: audible without stethoscope.

Signs of cardiac failure

● Resting tachycardia
● Elevation of the JVP (p. 20)
● Third or fourth heart sound (triple rhythm) (p. 25)
● Basal crepitations (p. 42)

- Hepatomegaly (p. 52)
- Dependent pitting oedema (p. 112)

Blood pressure

The patient should be sitting or lying comfortably and relaxed because anxiety and muscle contraction increase the blood pressure. Measurement of the blood pressure in the erect position should be undertaken in patients in whom postural hypotension requires to be excluded, e.g. autonomic neuropathy, hypotensive drug therapy, syncope. It is important to record the BP using a cuff of an appropriate size. In adults, a cuff with a bladder width of 12 cm and bladder length of 30–35 cm is usually satisfactory.

Examination sequence

❑ Place the centre of the inflatable cuff over the brachial artery and wind the cuff smoothly and firmly around the upper arm; check that the mercury column of the sphygmomanometer is at the same level as the arm cuff (Fig. 10).

❑ Locate the brachial pulse and inflate the cuff to just over systolic pressure, when the pulse is obliterated.

❑ Auscultate over the brachial artery while slowly reducing the pressure. The systolic pressure is when Korotkov sounds are

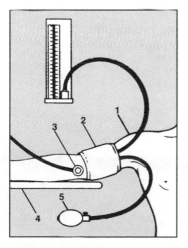

Fig. 10
Measurement of blood pressure. (1) no constricting garments; (2) apply cuff of the appropriate size; (3) palpate brachial pulse before applying stethoscope; (4) support arm at heart level; (5) inflate cuff until radial pulse is impalpable, check systolic pressure by auscultation, deflate slowly until diastolic pressure is reached.

first heard (phase 1) and the diastolic pressure, when sounds disappear (phase V).

Summary points

✦ Patients with significant cardiovascular disease may have no symptoms.
✦ Angina pectoris is typically induced by exertion and relieved by rest.
✦ The presence of nocturnal dyspnoea and orthopnoea are of limited value in helping to distinguish between cardiac and respiratory causes of breathlessness.
✦ The JVP provides important information and is the most reliable sign of cardiac failure.
✦ Auscultate the heart with the patient in the left semilateral position and then sitting or leaning forward to detect the murmurs of mitral and aortic regurgitation respectively.

The respiratory system

3

Cardinal symptoms

- Cough
- Sputum
- Haemoptysis
- Breathlessness
- Chest pain
- Wheeze
- Stridor

Enquiry should also be made about upper respiratory tract symptoms, such as nasal obstruction, bleeding and discharge, sore throat and hoarseness. Past and present smoking habits and any occupational hazard such as coal mining or exposure to asbestos should be noted.

○ **Cough** varies in nature depending on its cause. It may be harsh, dry and paroxysmal, loose and readily productive of sputum, or short and half-suppressed by pain. Cough may lack its normal explosive character when a vocal cord is paralysed (*'bovine' cough*).

○ **Sputum** may be *mucoid* (grey, white or 'clear'), *purulent* (yellow or green) or *mucopurulent* (a mixture of the two). If purulent, the amount of sputum produced may be of diagnostic importance, and the patient should be asked to estimate the daily volume.

○ **Haemoptysis** may range in amount from slight blood-staining of sputum to massive haemorrhage. Recurrent haemoptysis, even of slight degree, is often of greater significance than a single, major episode.

○ **Breathlessness (dyspnoea)** may be experienced only on exertion, or may occur in attacks when the patient is at rest. Non-respiratory causes of breathlessness include left heart failure, anaemia, obesity and anxiety. Exertional breathlessness should be assessed by asking about exercise tolerance; for example, 'How many flights of stairs can you climb without stopping?' The speed of onset and the duration of some respiratory causes of breathlessness may be of diagnostic significance (Table 3).

○ **Chest pain** caused by pulmonary disease is characteristically unilateral and aggravated by deep inspiration and coughing (*'pleuritic pain'*). Although this is usually localised to the chest wall, pain arising from the diaphragm is sometimes referred to the shoulder region or the anterior abdominal wall. Pain similar to that of pleurisy may be caused by disorders affecting the bones, muscles, nerves and joints of the chest wall and spine, and by pericarditis. Retrosternal discomfort not aggravated by respiration may be oesophageal in origin.

Table 3 Some respiratory causes of breathlessness	
Acute onset (hours/day)	Pulmonary embolism Pneumonia Acute asthma Pneumothorax
Intermediate (days/weeks)	Pleural effusion Bronchial carcinoma Pulmonary tuberculosis
Chronic (months/years)	Chronic obstructive pulmonary disease Pneumoconiosis Fibrosing alveolitis

○ **Wheeze** is a musical sound usually more conspicuous during expiration. It is almost invariably accompanied by dyspnoea, and is due to obstruction of the small airways.

○ **Stridor** is a '*crowing*' *sound* occurring during inspiration and aggravated by coughing; it is due to obstruction of the large airways (larynx or trachea).

PHYSICAL EXAMINATION

General observations

The examination of the respiratory system includes making a number of general observations for the presence or absence of such features as cyanosis and finger clubbing. The upper respiratory tract should not be overlooked although specialist equipment and expertise are required for the examination of the nasopharynx or larynx.

Examination sequence

❑ Inspect a specimen of sputum and confirm haemoptysis when present.

❑ Assess the nature of any cough, wheeze or stridor.

❑ Examine for finger clubbing (p. 114).

❑ Assess central cyanosis (p. 110).

❑ Examine for cervical lymphadenopathy in general and for scalene nodes in particular (p. 123).

❑ Inspect the mouth, teeth, pharynx and tonsils (p. 117).

❑ Press over each maxillary sinus to assess tenderness and compare one side with the other.

❑ Assess nasal airflow to exclude obstruction, one nostril at a time.

❑ Listen for stridor after asking the patient to cough.

Inspection

Physical examination of the chest consists of inspection, palpation, percussion and auscultation. The chest is inspected for lesions of the chest wall, abnormalities in the shape of the chest and the pattern and rate of respiration.

Examination sequence

❑ With the patient sitting, fully expose the evenly illuminated chest and upper abdomen.

❑ Minor asymmetry of the chest is sometimes best seen with the patient lying supine.

❑ When inspecting the back, the patient's arms should be folded across the chest.

❑ When inspecting the axillae, ask the patient to place the palms of the hands on the back of the head.

❑ Look for:
  • lesions of the chest wall
  • abnormalities of the shape of the chest
  • the mode of breathing
  • tracheal descent on inspiration (tracheal tug).

❑ Count the respiratory rate unobtrusively.

❑ Assess the degree and symmetry of movement on deep inspiration.

❑ Measure the maximum increase in chest expansion between inspiration and expiration using a tape measure around the chest at the level of the fourth or fifth rib.

The shape of the chest wall

In normal subjects, the ratio of the anteroposterior diameter of the chest relative to the lateral diameter is about 5 : 7. The A–P diameter is increased in emphysema (barrel chest).

Abnormalities of the shape of the chest wall

○ **Pectus carinatum** (*pigeon chest*) consists of a localised prominence of the sternum and adjacent costal cartilages (Fig. 11). It is often accompanied by indrawing of the ribs to form symmetrical horizontal grooves (*Harrison's sulci*) above everted costal margins. This may occur as a sequel to childhood asthma or rickets.

○ **Pectus excavatum** (*funnel chest*) is a developmental defect in

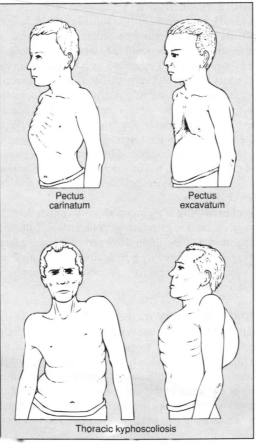

Pectus
carinatum

Pectus
excavatum

Thoracic kyphoscoliosis

**Fig. 11
Chest wall deformities.**

which there is a localised depression of the lower end of the sternum (Fig. 11) or, less commonly, depression of the whole length of the sternum and of the costal cartilages attached to it. This deformity may displace the heart but is usually asymptomatic.

○ **Thoracic kyphoscoliosis** (abnormal curvature of the spine) alters the position of the mediastinum in relation to the anterior chest wall, with the result that abnormalities in the position of the trachea and the apex beat may be mistakenly attributed to cardiac or pulmonary disease (Fig. 11). Asymmetry is an important sign if kyphoscoliosis is not present, as flattening implies underlying disease such as pulmonary fibrosis or collapse.

Respiratory movements

○ **Respiratory rate** is normally about 14 per minute in the adult.
○ **Respiratory depth** cannot be accurately measured by simple clinical assessment but it is possible to recognise marked degrees of hyper- or hypoventilation. The latter may be important in the diagnosis of ventilatory failure. Hyperventilation is due to stimulation of the respiratory centre as a result of anxiety, metabolic acidosis or head injury. *Periodic* or '*Cheyne–Stokes*' breathing is a cyclical variation in the depth of respiration, ranging from apnoea or hyperpnoea, due to decreased sensitivity of the respiratory centre to carbon dioxide. It occurs in left ventricular failure and brain stem ischaemia.
○ **Chest expansion** in a healthy person, i.e. the maximum difference in chest circumference between inspiration and expiration, should be 5 cm or more.
○ **Mode of breathing** is mainly abdominal rather than thoracic in normal subjects, and is effected by contraction of the diaphragm. Chest expansion may be limited by pleuritic pain; contraction of the diaphragm is restricted by peritonitis or abdominal distension. Normal expiration is a passive process and depends upon the elastic recoil of the lungs.

Abnormal respiratory movements

○ **Abnormal inspiratory movements.** Generalised indrawing of intercostal muscles occurs in patients who cannot achieve adequate ventilation by normal inspiratory efforts, e.g. when there is gross hyperinflation of the lungs in emphysema or asthma. Local indrawing of a portion of the chest wall during inspiration, '*paradoxical movements*', occurs in patients who have sustained double fractures of a series of ribs or of the sternum, and this may produce severe respiratory distress.
○ **Abnormal expiratory movements.** Powerful contractions of the abdominal muscles and latissimus dorsi are seen in asthma and

chronic bronchitis. Patients with severe airways obstruction may also be seen to exhale by puffing through pursed lips. This manoeuvre prevents collapse of the bronchial walls and minimises the work done during breathing.

○ **Asymmetry of movement.** Each side of the normal chest moves symmetrically. Reduced movement affecting part, or all, of one side is sometimes more obvious during deep breathing. When present, it is a strong indication of underlying disease.

Palpation

Palpation of the chest wall confirms the observations noted on inspection. Indeed, the symmetry of chest expansion is more readily assessed on inspection than by palpation. The position of the mediastinum can be assessed by palpating the trachea (Fig. 12) and locating the apex beat (p. 22).

Examination sequence

❏ Palpate any local abnormalities detected on inspection.

❏ Insert the tip of the index finger into the suprasternal notch in the midline to detect tracheal deviation; does the fingertip fit more easily into one or other side of the trachea? (Fig. 12).

❏ Measure the space in finger-breadths between the cricoid

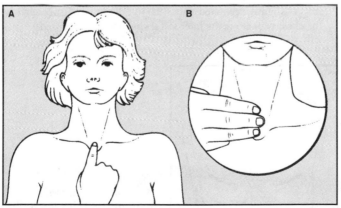

Fig. 12
A. Identifying the position of the trachea. B. Assessing the cricosternal distance.

cartilage and the suprasternal notch (the cricosternal distance) after the patient has made a full inspiration.

❏ Place both hands lightly on the anterior chest wall; assess the degree and symmetry of movement as the patient breathes in deeply by allowing the hands to separate as the chest expands. Repeat on the posterior chest wall (Fig. 13).

The trachea may be deviated towards the pathological side, for example in apical fibrosis or simple pneumothorax. Alternatively, it may be deviated away from the pathological side, for example in tension pneumothorax or large pleural effusion. *Subcutaneous emphysema* may be palpable as a 'crackling' sensation. Reduction in the *cricosternal distance* is a measure of the severity of obstructive airways disease. A low-pitched *rhonchus* or a *pleural rub* may sometimes be palpable.

Percussion

The subtle combination of changes in pitch and duration of the percussion note can be learned only by experience, but an immediate impression of the value of the sign can be gained by comparing the note over the lung, the liver and the stomach. The surface anatomy of the lung fields is shown in Figure 14.

Examination sequence

❏ Place the left hand on the chest wall, palm downwards with the fingers slightly separated. Press the middle finger firmly against the chest wall along the intercostal space to be percussed.

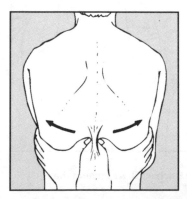

Fig. 13
Assessing respiratory movements of the lower ribs posteriorly; note that this is sometimes best assessed on inspection.

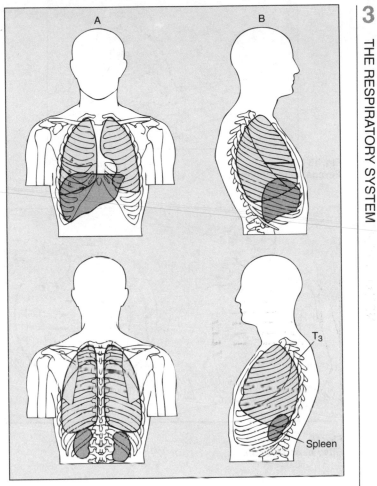

Fig. 14
Surface anatomy of the viscera: A. anterior and posterior;
B. lateral.

❑ Strike the centre of the middle phalanx of the middle finger
   sharply with the tip of the right middle finger. In order to
   produce a satisfactory percussion note, the right middle finger
   should be held in partial flexion and the entire movement
   should come from the wrist joint (Fig. 15).

❑ Compare the note at equivalent positions on the two sides.

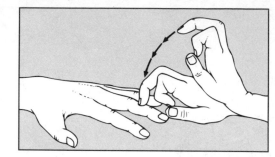

Fig. 15
Percussion technique.

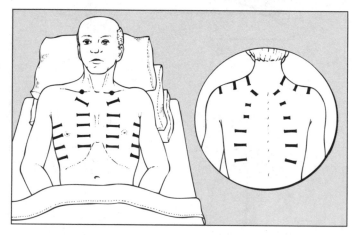

Fig. 16
Sites of percussion.

When an area of altered resonance is discovered, map out its
boundaries by percussing from a zone of normal resonance
towards the area of suspected abnormality.

❏ Percuss over the chest anteriorly, posteriorly and laterally and
over the apices of the upper lobes (Fig. 16).

Significance of changes in percussion note
The percussion note over normal lung is *resonant*. *Resonance* is
impaired or *dull* when the lung is separated from the chest wall by
pleural fluid or thickening, or pulmonary consolidation or collapse.

A characteristic *stony dull* note is elicited over a large pleural effusion. The area of dullness over the heart and liver is less extensive than would be expected from anatomical surface marking, since aerated lung is interposed. A *hyperresonant percussion note* may be found over a lung or part of a lung which is markedly emphysematous, and also over a large air-filled space, such as a pneumothorax. Below the diaphragm an underlying gas-containing viscus produces a *tympanitic note*.

Auscultation

Breath sounds

Breath sounds are produced by vibrations of the vocal cords caused by the flow of air through the larynx during inspiration and expiration. The sounds so produced are transmitted along the trachea and bronchi and through the lungs to the chest wall. These may be normal, vesicular, diminished vesicular, vesicular with prolonged expiration, or bronchial. Vesicular breath sounds are the normal sounds heard through a stethoscope applied to the chest over an area of aerated lung tissue. The intensity of these sounds increases steadily during inspiration and then quickly fades away during the first third of expiration.

Examination sequence

❑ Ask the patient to breathe in and out gently through the open mouth.

❑ Auscultate all over the chest wall to ensure that localised lesions are not overlooked.

❑ Compare the findings at equivalent positions on the two sides and remember to auscultate over the apices and in the axillae.

❑ Identify the intensity, quality and duration of breath sounds during inspiration and expiration.

❑ Note the site and character of any added sounds; check to see if the sound persists when the patient stops breathing.

❑ Assess vocal resonance by asking the patient to say 'ninety-nine' and compare the findings at equivalent positions on the two sides.

Significance of abnormalities on auscultation

Vesicular breath sounds are diminished in intensity if the chest wall is thick or if conduction of the sounds to the chest wall is reduced by shallow breathing, bronchial obstruction, emphysema, pneumothorax, pleural effusion or pleural thickening. The expiratory phase of vesicular breath sounds may be prolonged in the presence of airways obstruction, when it is often associated with expiratory rhonchi (see below). Bronchial breath sounds are heard when sounds produced in the larynx are transmitted via patent airways to the chest wall through lung tissue which has lost its normal consistency, thereby increasing sound conduction. Bronchial breath sounds are usually associated with pneumonic consolidation producing a uniform conducting medium, but may also be present in other conditions such as pulmonary fibrosis or cavitation. The finding of decreased rather than increased breath sounds over an area of consolidation strongly suggests obstruction of the corresponding major bronchus.

Criteria for bronchial breath sounds

- Both inspiratory and expiratory sounds are loud and blowing in character, similar to those heard over the trachea.
- The expiratory sound is as long and as loud as the inspiratory sound.
- There is an audible pause between the end of the inspiratory sound and the beginning of the expiratory sound.
- There is an increase in conduction of spoken and whispered sounds, *vocal resonance* and *whispering pectoriloquy* (p. 43).

Added sounds

These are of three different types:

- rhonchi (wheezes)
- crepitations (crackles)
- pleural rub (friction).

○ **Rhonchi** (wheezes) are musical sounds of high, medium or low pitch produced by the passage of air through narrowed bronchi. In asthma, rhonchi are predominantly high- and medium-pitched and expiratory, while in bronchitis they are usually medium- and low-pitched and are audible during both inspiration and expiration.

○ **Crepitations** (crackles) are non-musical sounds with a crackling quality. In some cases crepitations indicate excess secretions in the small airways. Such crepitations often increase in number temporarily after a short cough but may become less numerous or may disappear for a while after prolonged coughing. They are audible throughout inspiration. In other cases, crepitations are due to the explosive reopening, during inspiration, of peripheral airways which have been occluded during expiration by viscid exudate in the bronchioles or by thickening of the alveolar septa by oedema, inflammation or fibrosis. These crepitations are most numerous towards the end of inspiration and may be accompanied by rhonchi. They are not altered by coughing. Although a feature of pulmonary oedema, severe pulmonary oedema may occur in the absence of crepitations.

○ **A pleural rub** is a creaking sound produced by movement of the visceral over the parietal pleura when both surfaces have been roughened by a fibrinous exudate. It sounds like the crunching noise of footsteps in crisp snow or like the creaking of leather. It is usually audible at two separate stages of the respiratory cycle, towards the end of inspiration and just after the beginning of expiration. A pleural rub may be inaudible during quiet breathing but becomes easily heard when the patient takes a deep breath. In some cases a rub may be heard in the absence of pain, while in others severe pain may not be accompanied by a rub. Sometimes it may be difficult to distinguish between a low-pitched rhonchus and a pleural rub. After forceful coughing, rhonchi usually alter in character or disappear, while a pleural rub remains unchanged. The temptation to elicit a rub should be resisted when pleural pain is severe.

Voice resonance

Voice sounds are transmitted from the larynx to the chest wall and are modified in the same way as breath sounds, through the stethoscope, they normally have a muffled quality and are equal in intensity on the two sides. A localised reduction in breath sounds is accompanied by decreased voice sounds, for example over a pleural effusion. Bronchial breath sounds are accompanied by increased vocal resonance such that if the patient whispers, the sound is clearly audible, whispering pectoriloquy.

Interpretation of physical signs

A summary of the principal physical signs found in consolidation, collapse, pleural effusion, pneumothorax, emphysema and asthma is given in Table 4.

Summary points

✦ The degree of functional disability should be assessed in all
breathless patients.

Table 4
Typical signs in respiratory disorders

Abnormality	Chest wall movement	Mediastinal displacement	Percussion note	Breath sounds	Vocal resonance	Added sounds
Consolidation	Decreased on affected side	None	Dull	Bronchial	Increased	Crepitations
Collapse	Decreased on affected side	Towards affected side	Dull	Decreased or absent	Decreased or absent	None
Effusion	Decreased on affected side	Towards opposite side	Stony dull	Decreased or absent	Decreased or absent	May be a pleural rub
Pneumothorax	Decreased on affected side	Towards opposite side	Normal or hyperresonant	Decreased or absent	Decreased or absent	None
Emphysema	Decreased on both sides	None	Normal or hyperresonant	Decreased	Normal or decreased	None
Asthma	Decreased on both sides	None	Normal or hyperresonant	Prolonged expiration	Normal	Rhonchi

- Expiratory wheeze indicates small airways obstruction, and stridor, large airways obstruction.
- Bronchial breathing indicates the coexistence of a uniform conducting medium (often consolidation) and patent airways.
- Vocal resonance is a useful method of confirming the presence of bronchial breathing.
- Crepitations (crackles) which clear with coughing suggest fluid within the small airways.

The alimentary and genitourinary systems

4

Cardinal symptoms

- Loss of appetite
- Difficulty in swallowing
- Heartburn
- Abdominal pain
- Nausea
- Vomiting
- Weight loss
- Gastrointestinal bleeding
- Alteration in bowel habit
- Jaundice

Many such complaints may also be caused by disease in other systems; for example, epigastric pain may be due to acute myocardial infarction, vomiting may result from a cerebral tumour, and jaundice may be due to haemolysis.

○ **Anorexia** (loss of appetite) can occur in many systemic diseases and also in some psychological disorders. Local causes include gastric carcinoma and hepatitis.

○ **Dysphagia** (difficulty in swallowing) and *odynophagia* (pain on swallowing) should be regarded as symptoms which require a diagnosis and indicate oesophageal disease such as oesophagitis or carcinoma.

○ **Heartburn** is a retrosternal burning discomfort familiar to most healthy subjects and particularly common in pregnancy. It results from gastro-oesophageal reflux due to incompetence of the lower oesophageal sphincter.

○ **Abdominal pain** is an important symptom. Careful analysis often suggests the correct diagnosis; for example, duodenal ulceration causes pain which is usually localised to the epigastrium but may radiate to the back. It is gnawing in character and of moderate severity. The pain usually lasts for up to 2 hours but can be relieved within 15 minutes by eating or by antacids. It often occurs before meals and may waken the patient at night. The pain tends to be episodic, occurring two or three times daily for several weeks but with remissions lasting from weeks to months.

○ **Weight loss** may occur in any chronic wasting condition disorders such as malignancy, tuberculosis, thyrotoxicosis or uncontrolled diabetes mellitus. It is also a feature of anorexia nervosa. Weight loss is common in malabsorption syndromes and may be the presenting symptom of GI malignancy.

○ **Vomiting.** Important diagnostic features include details of the frequency and timing of vomiting, and its quantity, contents and colour together with the patient's opinion about the taste of the vomitus and pain relief after vomiting.

○ **Gastrointestinal haemorrhage.** The colour of the blood lost may indicate the source of bleeding. Bright red blood in the vomitus is usually oesophageal; bleeding from the stomach or duodenum results in a 'coffee-ground' appearance in the vomit. Significant upper GI haemorrhage produces black stools (*melaena*). Fresh blood in the stool occurs when the bleeding arises from the anorectum.

○ **Altered bowel habit.** Enquiry should be made as to the frequency, consistency and colour of the stool. Alteration in bowel habit may be an early symptom in colonic malignancy.

○ **Jaundice** associated with hepatitis or biliary obstruction causes dark urine and pale stools, but haemolytic jaundice does not because bilirubin is transported bound to albumin prior to its conjugation within the liver.

Symptoms of genitourinary disease

Many disorders of the kidneys do not cause local symptoms and may present with the features of renal failure or hypertension.

○ **Haematuria**, resulting from bleeding from the urinary tract, may be the only manifestation of serious disease of the urinary tract.

○ **Pain** is characteristically experienced in the back between the 12th rib and the iliac crest, loin pain, and may radiate in the dermatomes of the 12th thoracic and first lumbar spinal nerves. Severe, unremitting pain associated with nausea, vomiting and restlessness typifies obstruction of the renal pelvis and ureter and is called '*renal*' or '*ureteric colic*'. Burning pain (*dysuria*) and *frequency* of micturition may be caused by inflammation of the bladder or urethra.

○ **In the male**, *poor stream* (reduction in the force of the urinary stream), *urgency*, *hesitancy* and *dribbling incontinence* suggest bladder neck obstruction from prostatic disease.

○ **In the female**, urinary incontinence from coughing (*stress incontinence*) may follow trauma to the pelvic floor during childbirth and may be associated with *urge incontinence*, the inability to delay micturition following the call to void.

○ **Menstrual disorders** are common; *dysmenorrhoea* refers to painful menstruation (periods), *amenorrhoea* to the absence of periods and *polymenorrhoea* to an increased frequency of periods. A vaginal discharge suggests the presence of vaginal infection necessitating microbiological investigation.

○ **Vaginal bleeding** following sexual intercourse usually indicates local pathology such as a polyp, cervical erosion or malignancy.

○ **Sexual problems** in the male may present as *impotence* (erectile dysfunction), premature ejaculation or loss of sexual desire. In the female, loss of desire, inability to orgasm and pain on intercourse (*dyspareunia*) are the principal symptoms. Most sexual dysfunction has a psychological basis though occasionally physical causes such as diabetic autonomic neuropathy may explain the problem.

PHYSICAL EXAMINATION

Examination of the mouth and throat are described on page 117. The abdomen can be divided for descriptive purposes into nine regions by the intersection of two horizontal and two vertical planes (Fig. 17). Inspection and palpation constitute the main methods of examination of the abdomen, with percussion and auscultation fulfilling supplementary functions.

Palpation comprises light palpation, deep palpation and deep palpation during respiration. The liver, gall bladder, spleen and kidneys move with respiration. In the normal abdomen it may be possible to feel the lower edge of the liver, the lower pole of the right kidney, a distended bladder, the aorta, faeces in the descending colon and the gravid uterus (Fig. 18). The main value of abdominal percussion is to decide whether distension is due to gas, fluid (*ascites*) or a cystic or solid tumour. Auscultation is performed to listen for bowel sounds, vascular bruits and, occasionally, hepatic and splenic friction rubs.

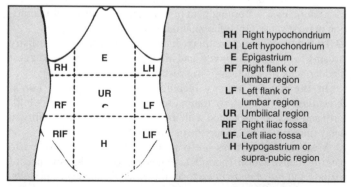

Fig. 17
Regions of the abdomen.

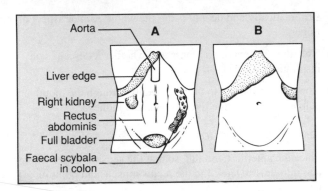

Labels for figure A (top to bottom): Aorta, Liver edge, Right kidney, Rectus abdominis, Full bladder, Faecal scybala in colon

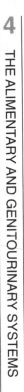

Fig. 18
Abdominal palpation. A. Findings which may be normal.
B. Hepatosplenomegaly.

Examination sequence

General observations

❑ Examine the patient in a good light and in warm surroundings.

❑ Position the patient comfortably, lying supine with the head on a pillow and the arms by the sides as this helps to relax the abdominal muscles.

❑ Expose the skin from the xiphisternum to the symphysis pubis.

❑ Observe the general shape and symmetry of the abdomen; ask the patient to identify any scars, and note any changes in the skin or hair, abnormal veins, pulsations or movements.

❑ Stand, sit or kneel comfortably beside the patient.

❑ Ask the patient to report any discomfort and watch the patient's face for signs of discomfort.

Palpation

❑ Use warm hands to palpate the abdomen.

❑ Begin palpation in an area remote from the site of any pain.

❑ Use light palpation to test muscle tone, using gentle dipping movements as the hand is moved from region to region without breaking contact with the skin.

❑ With the patient breathing naturally, palpate the abdomen

systematically and deeply using the whole palmar aspect of the fingers.

❑ Note the features of any mass and whether it descends on inspiration (p. 123).

❑ Now ask the patient to breathe deeply through the mouth and palpate in turn for the liver, spleen and kidneys.

Liver and gall bladder

❑ Place the anterior hand flat, so that the sensing fingers (index and middle) are lateral to the rectus muscle and pointing upwards (Fig. 19).

❑ Push the hand slightly inwards and upwards until, at the height of inspiration, the former pressure is released, allowing the fingers to slip over the edge of a palpable liver.

❑ Move the fingers towards the costal margin with each inspiration until the liver edge becomes palpable.

❑ Move the hand medially to trace the liver edge across the abdomen. Note its shape, size, consistency and any tenderness.

❑ Ask the patient to breathe in deeply while palpating over the gall bladder; look for tenderness and identify the gall bladder if palpable.

Spleen

❑ Lay the front hand flat with the fingers at right angles to the left costal margin and press inwards and upwards (Fig. 19).

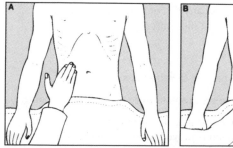
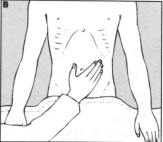

Fig. 19
Palpation of the liver/spleen **A.** Liver. **B.** Spleen.

- After each inspiration, move the anterior hand upwards until the fingertips are under the costal margin.

- Repeat the process along the rib margin, as the position of the spleen tip varies.

Kidneys

- Use bimanual palpation to examine the kidneys.

- Place the posterior hand in the renal angle and, with the fingers pressed forwards, position the anterior hand along the horizontal plane with the fingertips over the rectus muscle (Fig. 20).

- Using gentle but deep palpation, bring the two hands as close together as possible while the patient breathes deeply.

- The kidney may be felt to descend and sometimes may even be caught between the two hands. When the pressure is released, the kidney will slide upwards on expiration.

- The left kidney can be examined from either side of the patient (Fig. 20).

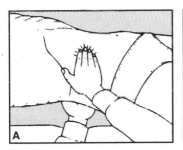

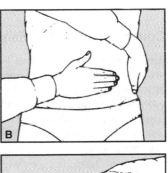

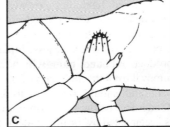

Fig. 20
Palpation of the kidneys.
A. Right kidney from right side.
B. Left kidney from right side.
C. Left kidney from left side.

Percussion

❏ Percuss from resonant to dull.

❏ Place the finger parallel to the line of anticipated change of note.

❏ Percuss deeply for deep structures (e.g. upper border of the liver), and more lightly for superficial structures.

❏ When eliciting '*shifting dullness*', percuss towards the flank until a dull note is obtained.
— Without moving the hand, roll the patient onto the opposite side and wait for the fluid to redistribute.
— Percuss again; if the note is resonant, confirm the finding by percussing back towards the midline, where a dull note will be present.

❏ To elicit a gastric *succussion splash*, shake the patient vigorously from side to side.

Auscultation

❏ Listen for bowel sounds for at least 1 minute.

❏ Identify vascular bruits, and listen over the liver and spleen for any friction rubs.

Common abnormalities

Any asymmetry, skin lesions and abnormal pulsations should be noted. Epigastric pulsations usually arise from the abdominal aorta or are transmitted from the heart. Pyloric obstruction can cause visible gastric peristalsis. Slow waves passing from the left sub-costal area to and across the midline are most easily observed on tangential inspection. Small bowel peristalsis is seen as writhing movements in the central abdomen.

Localised tenderness or rigidity is usually associated with organic disease. Generalised rigidity commonly implies failure of the patient to relax but is also a feature of peritonitis, when it is accompanied by tenderness. Inflammation of the peritoneum will produce rebound pain which can be elicited by the sudden removal from the abdomen of the firmly applied hand. This causes pain and should only be looked for in doubtful situations. Tenderness below the midpoint of the right costal margin which is accentuated by, or limits, deep inspiration suggests acute cholecystitis (*Murphy's sign*). Acute appendicitis is often associated with tenderness over an area a third of the way between the right superior iliac spine and the umbilicus (*McBurney's point*). Renal tenderness is usually most marked posteriorly.

Enlargement of the liver may be a feature of cardiac failure, hepatitis or disseminated malignancy. Palpable enlargement of the gall bladder suggests either obstruction of the cystic duct, in which case the patient will not be jaundiced, or of the common bile duct, when there is jaundice. Enlargement of one kidney may occur with renal carcinoma, hydronephrosis or compensatory hypertrophy following damage to the other kidney. Bilateral renal enlargement is a feature of polycystic renal disease. The spleen is only palpable if considerably enlarged. This may occur with various infections such as malaria or glandular fever, myeloproliferative diseases and in portal hypertension.

The spleen can be distinguished from the left kidney most readily by the fact that it is possible to insert the fingers beneath and round the lower pole of the spleen. It is impossible to do this with the kidney unless a mass is projecting from it, which is rare. Other features are the inability to place the hand between the spleen and rib cage, and the fact that marked splenic enlargement tends to occur in both a downward and a medial direction. A notch is palpable on the medial border only when the spleen extends several centimetres below the costal margin.

Gaseous distension and swellings overlaid by gas will be resonant. With ascites, gut containing gas floats uppermost, while the fluid accumulates in both flanks when the patient is lying supine; when the patient lies on one or other side, the ascites accumulates there. In contrast, pelvic masses extending into the abdomen cause displacement of bowel to the flanks, resulting in central dullness on percussion with resonance in the flanks. Percussion is a poor method of confirming enlargement of the liver, but may be helpful in defining a distended bladder, an ovarian cyst or a degree of splenomegaly which cannot be detected on palpation. A gastric *succussion splash* can normally be elicited 1–2 hours after eating or drinking. If present several hours after a meal, it suggests the presence of gastric outlet obstruction.

Normal peristaltic activity produces characteristic gurgling sounds which can be heard with the stethoscope every 5–10 seconds. Bowel sounds occur more frequently when peristalsis is increased by gastroenteritis, by the effects of blood in gut or by *mechanical obstruction*; in obstruction, bowel sounds have a high-pitched tinkling character. The sounds disappear when the bowel is rendered inactive (*paralytic ileus*), as in generalised peritonitis.

Aortic bruits may occur in healthy subjects, or bruits may arise from stenotic lesions in the aorta, mesenteric or renal arteries. Hepatic bruits can occur in alcoholic liver disease and liver tumours. Friction rubs may occasionally be heard over inflammatory and neoplastic disease of the liver and infarcts of the spleen.

Examination of the groins and hernial orifices

The groins should be examined for external hernias and lymph nodes. Lymph nodes of up to 1 centimetre in diameter are often present in health.

Examination sequence

❏ With the patient lying supine, examine for inguinal lymph nodes.

❏ Ask the patient to stand, inspect the inguinal and femoral canals and the scrotum for hernias; ask the patient to cough and observe any impulse in the inguinal canals and/or scrotum.

❏ Invaginate the scrotum with the little finger and gently palpate the external inguinal ring and posterior wall of the inguinal canal for possible muscle defects.

❏ Feel for any impulse as the patient coughs; if a hernia is present, attempt to reduce the hernia by applying gentle, sustained pressure and by 'massaging' the hernia towards the internal ring.

❏ Once the hernia is reduced, occlude the internal inguinal ring with finger pressure at the mid-inguinal point and check to see if the hernia reappears during coughing.

❏ Identify the anatomical relationships between the hernia, the pubic tubercle and the inguinal ligament to distinguish femoral hernias from inguinal hernias.

Pathological lymph nodes are usually enlarged and may be matted together and feel firmer than normal glands. Inguinal and femoral hernias can best be distinguished by their relationships to the pubic tubercle and inguinal ligament; inguinal hernias lie above and medial to the pubic tubercle and femoral hernias, below and lateral to the pubic tubercle. Inguinal hernias, unlike femoral hernias, usually transmit an impulse on coughing but not if the hernia is strangulated.

Examination of male genitalia

Examination of the testes is particularly important in acute abdominal pain as torsion of the testis can cause abdominal pain and delayed diagnosis can result in orchidectomy.

Examination sequence

❑ Examine the penis and carefully palpate the testes, epididymes and vasa deferentia.

❑ Examine the scrotum and palpate both testes to determine the exact site of any swelling (Fig. 21).

❑ Confirm that any swelling originates in the scrotum and is not an inguinal hernia.

❑ Use a pen torch to transilluminate any scrotal swelling to see if it is cystic.

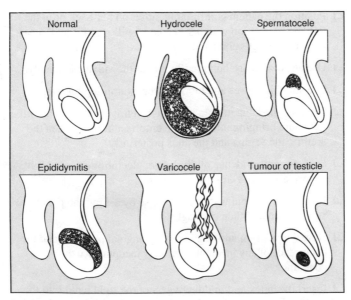

Fig. 21
Swellings of the scrotum.

Any scrotal swelling should be examined using the principles outlined on page 123. A hydrocele can usually be transilluminated and can be differentiated from a spermatocele and a cyst of the epididymis by its relationship to the testis. The possibility that a hydrocele may obscure a testicular tumour should not be overlooked and in each case the testis should be palpated with care.

Examination of the female genitalia

Vaginal examination is not routine. Its intimate nature raises medicolegal considerations necessitating both informed consent and the presence of a chaperone. The vaginal examination of females with an intact hymen should be avoided particularly as the information required can often be obtained by digital examination of the rectum. Vaginal examination of a minor requires the consent of a parent or guardian.

Examination sequence

❑ Ask the patient to empty the bladder before beginning the examination.

❑ Position the patient comfortably either on her back or in the left lateral position with her head on a pillow, hips and knees flexed and thighs abducted.

❑ Use an Anglepoise lamp to illuminate the vulva adequately.

❑ Use suitable gloves and lubricate the examining fingers.

❑ Separate the labia minora with the forefinger and thumb of the left hand, bringing into view the clitoris anteriorly, then the urethra, the vagina and the anus posteriorly.

❑ Look for any evidence of discharge, ulceration or abnormalities of Bartholin's glands.

❑ Inspect the vaginal walls for prolapse by asking the patient to strain down and then to cough.

❑ Note the position and degree of any vaginal prolapse and the occurrence of any involuntary urinary incontinence on coughing.

❑ Insert the index and middle fingers of the right hand into the vagina and rotate palm-upwards. Use only one finger if vaginismus or atrophic vaginitis makes examination painful.

- ❏ Palpate the cervix; the normal cervix points downwards and slightly backwards and feels like the tip of the nose.
- ❏ Note any tenderness on movement of the cervix (*cervical excitation*).
- ❏ Now perform bimanual palpation; with two fingers in the anterior fornix, place the left hand flat on the abdomen above the pubis.
- ❏ Identify the size, position and surface characteristics of the uterus between the hands.
- ❏ If the uterus is not palpable, palpate with the fingers in the posterior fornix as the uterus may be retroverted.
- ❏ Palpate each lateral fornix in turn bimanually.
- ❏ Note any tenderness or swelling of the fallopian tubes or ovaries (*adnexae*), the bladder anteriorly and the pouch of Douglas posteriorly.

Digital examination of the rectum

Many errors in diagnosis have been made because examination of the rectum has been omitted. The patient, chaperoned if necessary, should be informed of the need to examine the back passage. The presence of an anal fissure renders digital examination of the rectum very painful. If painful anorectal disease is suspected, digital examination should only be undertaken after applying local anaesthetic gel to the anal canal; a general anaesthetic, however, may be required.

Examination sequence

- ❏ Place the patient in the left lateral position with the buttocks at the edge of the couch, the knees drawn up to the chest and the heels clear of the perineum.
- ❏ Reassure the patient and explain that the examination may be uncomfortable but should not be painful.
- ❏ Lubricate the examining index finger, protected by a suitable glove.
- ❏ Examine the perianal skin in a good light looking for evidence of skin lesions, external haemorrhoids or fistulae.
- ❏ Place the tip of the forefinger on the anal margin and with

steady pressure on the sphincter pass the finger gently through the anal canal into the rectum.

❏ If anal spasm is encountered, ask the patient to breathe out and relax. If the patient experiences a significant degree of anal pain, do not proceed further but seek advice.

❏ Ask the patient to squeeze the examining forefinger with the anal sphincter.

❏ Note any weakness of sphincter contraction.

❏ Palpate around the entire rectum.

❏ Note any abnormality and examine any mass systematically.

❏ Note the percentage of the rectal circumference involved by disease and the distance of the upper and lower edges of disease from the anal canal.

❏ Perform bimanual examination if necessary, using the other hand laid flat over the lower abdomen.

❏ Repeat the examination after the patient has defecated if in doubt about palpable masses.

❏ After withdrawal, examine the finger for stool colour and the presence of blood and mucus.

❏ Test the stool sample for blood using a 'Haemoccult' testing card.

The rectum is normally empty and the walls smooth and soft. Posteriorly, the coccyx and sacrum can be felt through the rectal wall. In the female, the firm round cervix uteri can be felt anteriorly (Fig. 22C); the presence of a vaginal tampon or pessary may also be felt and may cause confusion. In the male the prostate is readily felt anteriorly (Fig. 22D). The normal prostate gland is smooth and has a firm consistency, with the contours of miniature buttocks represented by a shallow median groove between the lateral lobes. Haemorrhoids which are not thrombosed and normal seminal vesicles cannot be felt.

Proctoscopy

Visual examination of the rectum and anal canal is essential for the diagnosis of inflammatory lesions and haemorrhoids. Through the proctoscope, the surface of the normal rectum is similar in appearance to that of buccal mucosa: clean, shiny, smooth and reddish-pink but with clearly visible submucosal veins. Haemorrhoids and

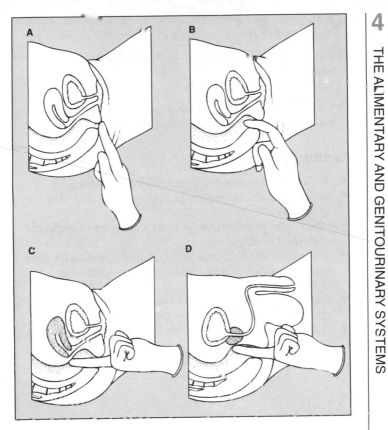

Fig. 22
Examination of the rectum. The finger is placed on the external
sphincter **A.** and inserted into the rectum **B.** The hand is then rotated
and the most prominent features are the cervix in the female **C.** and the
prostate in the male **D.**

rectal prolapse are more readily detected when the patient strains
downwards as the proctoscope is slowly withdrawn.

Examination sequence

❑ With the patient in the left lateral position, separate the
buttocks with the forefinger and thumb of one hand and with
the other hand gently insert a well-lubricated proctoscope with
obdurator in the direction of the umbilicus, through the anal
canal into the rectum.

❑ Remove the obturator and examine the rectal mucosa carefully under good illumination, noting any abnormality seen.

❑ Ask the patient to strain down as the instrument is slowly withdrawn to detect any degree of rectal prolapse and the severity of any haemorrhoids.

❑ Carefully examine the anal canal for fissures, particularly if the patient has experienced pain during the procedure.

Summary points

✦ Vomiting and/or dysphagia require an explanation.

✦ Severe renal disease may be present in the absence of urinary symptoms or signs.

✦ Observe the patient's face for signs of discomfort during the abdominal examination.

✦ The patient should breathe deeply during palpation for those organs which move with respiration (liver, spleen and kidneys).

✦ Superficial palpation is often a successful method of detecting splenomegaly and/or hepatomegaly.

✦ The spleen is not palpable unless it is considerably enlarged.

The nervous system 5

HISTORY

Cardinal symptoms

- Headache
- Dizziness
- Blackout
- Visual impairment
- Deafness
- Paraesthesiae
- Weakness
- Sphincter dysfunction

Symptom patterns and the pathological process

It is important to ascertain the precise meaning of patients' symptoms and the terms used to describe them. Only after carefully listening to their own account of the illness should specific questions be asked about other neurological symptoms. The neurological history should record in detail the nature and course of symptoms in terms of their time–intensity relationships. In this way, the pattern of symptoms can be interpreted more easily. For example, sudden neurological defects suggest a vascular disorder; a chronic history of relapsing symptoms with anatomically unrelated physical signs suggest a demyelinating disorder. Chronic but progressive disorders suggest degenerative, metabolic or neoplastic disorders. In patients with neurological disease, it is often possible to make a firm diagnosis on clinical grounds alone though confirmation may require further investigation.

○ **Headache** should be analysed as for any other pain (p. 5). Headache is often caused by nervous tension, but when due to an expanding intracranial lesion it may be associated with vomiting, focal symptoms or impairment of consciousness.

○ **Dizziness**, *giddiness* or *lightheadedness* require clarification as the patient may have experienced one or more of the following:

- Loss of balance with an accompanying sense of rotation (*vertigo*)
- Loss of coordination as if about to fall
- Falling to the ground without loss of consciousness
- Feeling as if about to faint (*presyncope*)
- Feeling anxious and panicky.

○ **Blackout** (*unconsciousness*) may be sudden in onset and without warning or gradual in onset and heralded by feeling faint and lightheaded. Patients who lose consciousness while standing, as distinct from patients who fall, do not remember even hitting the ground. Description of events by an eye-witness should be obtained whenever possible, e.g. the loss of facial colour and absence of the pulse help to distinguish cardiac syncope from epilepsy.

○ **Visual impairment** may comprise *photophobia* (intolerance of light), *photopsia* (seeing flashes and zigzags of light), *diplopia* (double vision), *amblyopia* (blurred vision), loss of part of the field of vision of one eye (*scotoma*), *hemianopia*, loss of half of the field of vision of both eyes or *quadrantanopia*, loss of one-quarter of the field of vision of both eyes. Episodes of diplopia and blurred vision are common in multiple sclerosis. A transient visual disorder may be a typical prelude to a migrainous headache.

○ **Deafness** is common with advancing age and minor degrees are often overlooked. *Tinnitus*, a buzzing or ringing in the ears, when associated with deafness, suggests inner ear disease.

○ **Paraesthesiae** (tingling or numbness) are due to involvement of sensory pathways between the peripheral nerve endings up to and including, the parietal cortex.

○ **Weakness** may be due to a disorder of the upper or lower motor neurone, myoneural junction or muscle. It may be proximal, distal or global in extent.

○ **Sphincter dysfunction** more frequently involves bladder function than bowel function. Bladder sensory loss leads to painless urinary retention with overflow. Bladder motor loss usually causes urgency with impaired voluntary initiation of micturition. Combined sensory and motor loss due to spinal cord lesions produces an autonomous bladder with reflex bladder emptying.

PHYSICAL EXAMINATION

The detailed neurological examination is often begun with an assessment of the patient's ability to communicate (*speech and language functions*), intellect (*cognitive function*) and gait (p. 103). Once the general assessment has been completed, motor system, sensory system, peripheral reflexes and cranial nerves should be examined. In patients who are seriously ill or in pain, it may be advisable to begin with the assessment of the obvious abnormalities and, if necessary, defer the rest of the examination until later.

Speech

○ **Dysphasia.** Impairment of language function, may be *expres-*

sive (motor), when patients understand what is said and know what they wish to say but are unable to say it. It is *receptive* (sensory) when there is impairment of comprehension. Often there is a combination of receptive and expressive defects, *global dysphasia*. Inability to understand written language is termed *dyslexia*. Disorders of language arise from lesions of the speech areas in the dominant hemisphere.

○ **Dysarthria.** Speech may be normal in its use of language, but impaired because of difficulty in articulation (*dysarthria*) owing to defective movements of lips, tongue or palate. Dysarthria may be caused by diseases of the cerebellum or its connections when the speech becomes scanning or staccato, or by diseases of the motor neurones when the words become slurred and indistinct.

○ **Dysphonia.** Abnormalities of speech may also arise from impairment of sound production, *dysphonia*, usually due to vocal cord lesions, neuromuscular weakness or extrapyramidal disorders of basal ganglia or cerebellum.

Examination sequence

❏ Ask the patient to perform commands of increasing complexity, e.g. 'Close your eyes and open your mouth' (sensory dysphasia).

❏ Ask the patient to repeat a simple sentence *verbatim* and then to describe everyday procedures, e.g. making a cup of tea (motor dysphasia).

❏ Ask the patient to read aloud (dyslexia) and to repeat words containing labial and lingual consonants, as in 'British constitution' and 'artillery' (dysarthria).

❏ Ask the patient to write down his or her name and address (global language dysfunction).

Intellectual function

Identifying impairment of cognitive function requires awareness of the patient's normal intelligence. This may best be assessed by talking to a close relative or friend. It is important to ask the patient questions that are relevant to the patient's social background and to which the examiner knows the answer. Not knowing the result of a recent local football match may indicate severe impairment in one patient and normal function in another.

Examination sequence

❑ Assess orientation in time and place by asking the year, month, day of the week, time of day and place of interview.

❑ Test memory by the patient's ability to recall both recent and distant events.

❑ Test attention and concentration using the '*serial sevens*' *test*. Ask the patient to subtract 7 from 100 and to continue to subtract 7 from the remainder. (The test should normally be completed within 1 minute with no more than two mistakes.)

❑ Test general knowledge by asking relevant questions about current affairs or events.

❑ Assess intelligence from patients' accounts of themselves, their occupation and capacity to reason.

❑ Ask the patient to explain the meaning of common proverbs such as 'every cloud has a silver lining' or 'a stitch in time saves nine'.

The *Abbreviated Mental Test* (AMT) can be used to assess the degree of intellectual impairment.

Abbreviated Mental Test
(Score 1 for each correct response.)

- How old are you?
- What is your date of birth?
- What day of the week is it today?
- What month is this?
- What year is this?
- Remember the following address (e.g. 42 West Street).
- What is the name of this place, where we are now?
- What year was the start of World War II?
- What is the name of the present monarch?
- Count backwards from 20 to 1. (Score 0 for any uncorrected error.)
- Repeat the address I asked you to remember.

Normal score: 8+
Mild–moderate dementia: 4–7
Moderate–severe dementia: <4

EXAMINATION OF THE MOTOR SYSTEM

The motor pathways are shown in Figure 23.

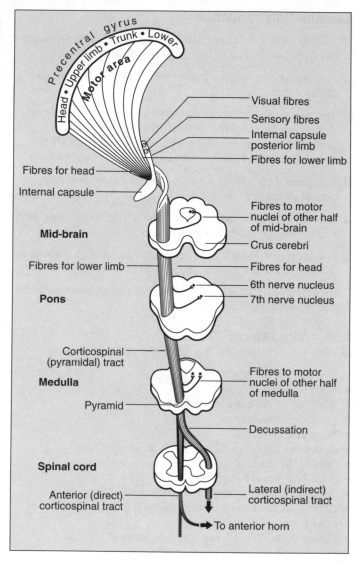

Fig. 23
The motor pathways.

Inspection

○ **Muscle wasting** is common in conditions associated with physical inactivity; it is more suggestive of an abnormality when it is asymmetrical rather than symmetrical.

○ **Fasciculation** refers to visible muscle twitching which occurs randomly at rest and stops during voluntary movements; it suggests a lesion in the proximal part of the lower motor neurones.

Involuntary movements

○ **Tremors** result from alternate contraction and relaxation of groups of muscles producing rhythmic oscillations about a joint or group of joints. There are three types of tremor:

• *Action tremor* is the commonest tremor and is an exaggeration of the 10-cycles-per-second physiological tremor which underlies all apparently smooth movements. An increase in physiological tremor is often found in anxiety, hyperthyroidism and alcohol withdrawal.

• *Resting tremor* is a coarser, slower tremor of 5 cycles per second; it is maximal at rest but absent during sleep, reduced during voluntary movement and increased by emotion. Typically it occurs in parkinsonism often producing adduction–abduction movements of the thumb with flexion and extension movements of the fingers.

• *Intention tremor* is a coarse, slow tremor of 5 cycles per second which is maximal during movement and absent at rest; it is characteristic of cerebellar disorders.

○ **Choreiform movements** are irregular, jerky, ill-sustained and appear semi-purposive. They affect different muscles unpredictably.

○ **Athetoid movements** are slow, writhing movements of the distal parts of the limbs particularly.

○ **Myoclonus** comprises sudden, shock-like movements of a whole limb, common in healthy subjects when falling asleep.

○ **Tics** are repetitive, localised and jerky.

Parkinsonian, choreiform and athetoid movements are caused by lesions of the basal ganglia.

Tone

Tone, the resistance felt when a joint is moved passively, is best assessed with the patient relaxed, neither assisting nor resisting passive limb movements.

○ **Hypertonia** (increased tone) is of two distinct types: spasticity and rigidity.

• *Spasticity* indicates pyramidal tract disorders of the upper motor neurones and produces an increasing resistance to the first few degrees of passive movement, then, as the movement continues, there is a sudden lessening of resistance (*'clasp knife' spasticity*).

● *Rigidity* indicates extrapyramidal tract disorders of the basal ganglia and produces a sustained resistance throughout the range of movement (*'lead-pipe' rigidity*). *'Cogwheel' rigidity* is the jerky resistance to passive movement seen in Parkinson's disease which results from the combination of a parkinsonian tremor and rigidity; it is often most apparent at the wrist joint.

○ **Hypotonia** (decreased tone) is more difficult to assess unless the lesion is unilateral, when comparison can be made with the normal side. Hypotonia occurs in disorders of the lower motor neurone and cerebellum; it is also sometimes present during the first few days after the sudden onset of upper motor neurone damage.

Power

Occasionally all muscle groups require assessment; usually this is not necessary. The power in the upper limbs is normally greater on the dominant side.

○ **Isometric testing** involves the patient attempting to maintain a limb position whilst the examiner tries to move the limb.

○ **Isotonic testing** is a more sensitive method; the patient attempts specific limb movements while the examiner opposes the movement.

Muscle power can be usefully assessed using the MRC scale (Table 5). The inability to perform fine, coordinated finger movements is typically found at an early stage in both pyramidal and extrapyramidal tract disorders.

Table 5 MRC muscle power scale	
Grade 0	No muscle contraction visible
Grade 1	Muscle contraction visible but no movement
Grade 2	Movement when the effect of gravity eliminated
Grade 3	Movement sufficient to overcome gravity
Grade 4	Movement to overcome gravity plus added resistance
Grade 5	Normal power

Examination sequence

General inspection

❑ Inspect the shape and bulk of the patient's musculature and note any asymmetry.

❏ Look for spontaneous fasciculation, especially in the deltoids, thighs and calves.

❏ Look for any involuntary movements and identify their nature.

❏ Assess the rate and amplitude of any tremor and the effect of movement on tremor.

❏ Look for a tremor as the patient maintains the hands and arms in the outstretched position.

Tone

❏ Ask the patient to relax in the supine position and to let the limbs go loose and floppy.

❏ Flex and extend the limbs at the wrists, elbows, knees and hips; at first, manipulate each joint slowly then more rapidly.

❏ Assess tone at the wrist by shaking the forearm and observing the hand.

❏ Assess tone at the ankle by rolling the leg to and fro and observing the foot.

Power

❏ Check whether the patient is right- or left-handed.

❏ Assess the power in the limbs both proximally and distally.

❏ Compare one muscle group with the same group on the other side.

Fine movements

❏ Ask the patient to make 'piano-playing' finger movements with both arms outstretched.

❏ Observe the patient performing everyday activities such as fastening buttons or tying knots.

EXAMINATION OF THE REFLEXES

○ **The reflex arc** consists of an afferent pathway triggered by stimulating a receptor, an efferent system which activates an

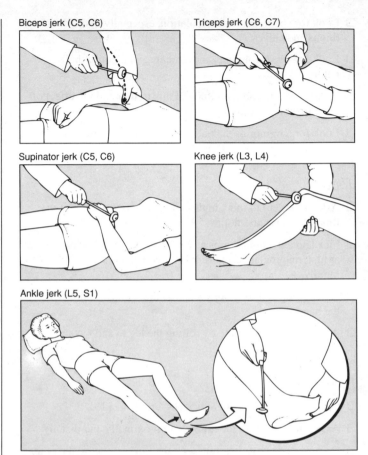

Fig. 24
Eliciting tendon reflexes (principal segmental innervations).

effector organ and a communication between these two components. Since reflex responses are involuntary and any interruption of the reflex arc will result in loss or diminution of the reflex, disturbances of the reflexes provide strong evidence of neurological dysfunction. Neurological examination should include the common tendon and cutaneous reflexes.

Tendon reflexes

Supinator (C5–C6), biceps (C5–C6), triceps (C6–C7), knee (L3–L4) and ankle reflexes (L5–S1) are evoked by a brisk stretch of the appropriate tendon using a tendon hammer. The tendon, not the muscle, should be struck, as stimulation of a muscle belly produces a contraction which is independent of the reflex arc. Tendon reflexes may be normal, increased, decreased, absent or exhibit delayed muscle relaxation. *Clonus* is the rhythmic repetition of involuntary muscular contractions evoked by a sudden passive stretch of a muscle. A few beats of clonus elicited in anxious patients may not be significant.

Examination sequence

❑ Place the patient in a comfortably relaxed position to facilitate easy access to the limbs (Fig. 24).

❑ Identify the tendon by palpation and then tap it with a tendon hammer, using a swinging motion from the wrist.

❑ Compare the reflex responses on both sides, noting any delay in muscle relaxation or asymmetry of response.

❑ If no reflex is observed, repeat using reinforcement:
  - In the upper limbs, ask the patient to clench the jaws or squeeze the knees together just before the tendon is struck, and then to relax
  - In the lower limbs, ask the patient to lock the two hands together and to attempt to pull them apart just before the tendon is struck, then to relax (Fig. 25).

Hoffmann reflex

❑ Flex the distal interphalangeal joint of the patient's middle finger between your finger and thumb.

❑ Withdraw thumb pressure abruptly to 'flick' the distal phalanx into extension.

❑ Look for reflex flexion of the thumb and forefinger.

Clonus

❑ In a relaxed patient in the supine position with the knee extended, push the patella down briskly towards the foot to elicit knee clonus (Fig. 26A).

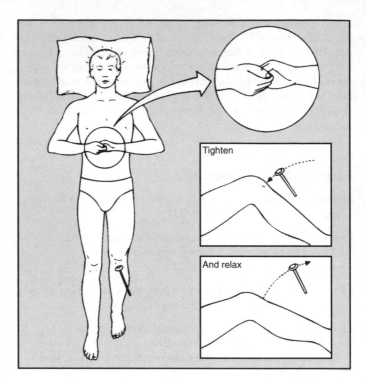

Fig. 25
Reinforcing the knee jerk.

❑ With the knees flexed and the ankle in a neutral position, dorsiflex the foot briskly to elicit ankle clonus (Fig. 26B).

Increased tendon reflexes

Upper motor neurone lesions produce pathologically brisk tendon reflexes. Reflexes may be increased as a result of anxiety; whether a reflex is abnormally brisk may therefore depend upon the presence of other features of *hyperreflexia*. For example, hyperreflexia in the upper limbs is suggested by the presence of a Hoffmann reflex and in the lower limbs, by sustained clonus (i.e. contractions which continue as long as stretch is applied) and is confirmed by the presence of extensor plantar responses (see below).

Decreased or absent tendon reflexes

The significance of depressed tendon reflexes requires careful appraisal because they may be difficult to elicit in some healthy

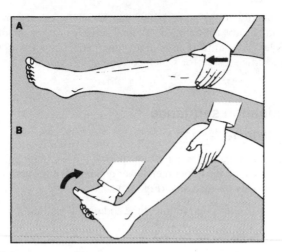

Fig. 26
Testing for knee and ankle clonus.

subjects. However, the absence of one or more tendon reflexes especially if asymmetrical usually denotes a lower motor neurone lesion. When no response is obtained, the absence of the reflex should be confirmed by '*reinforcement*'.

○ **Delayed muscle relaxation** is characteristic of hypothermia and hypothyroidism and is usually most easily demonstrable in the ankle jerk.

Superficial reflexes

These consist of muscle contractions evoked in response to cutaneous stimulation. The plantar response is the best known and most important.

Plantar reflex (L5–S1)

Except in infancy, stimulation of the sole of the foot normally produces plantar flexion of the great toe and usually of the other toes. A lesion of the upper motor neurone causes dorsiflexion of the great toe and often a fanning of the other toes; this is known as the *extensor plantar response* (*Babinski's sign*). Absent plantar responses may simply indicate cold feet.

Abdominal reflexes (T6–T12)

Normally, stroking the skin of the anterior abdominal wall induces a contraction of the underlying muscles. The reflexes may be absent in obesity, following abdominal surgery or if the abdominal wall is lax. Absent responses in a young patient suggest an upper motor neurone lesion for which corroborative evidence should be sought.

Examination sequence

Abdominal reflexes

❑ In a relaxed patient in the supine position, use a blunt point to lightly scrape the upper then lower quadrants of the abdominal wall swiftly on each side (Fig. 27A).

❑ Look for reflex contraction of the abdominal wall muscles.

Plantar reflex

❑ In a relaxed patient in the supine position, slowly draw a blunt point, such as the examiner's thumbnail, along the lateral border of the foot from the heel towards the little toe (Fig. 27B).

❑ Record the direction of the initial movement of the great toe and look for fanning of the toes. Stop as soon as movement occurs and avoid undue repetition.

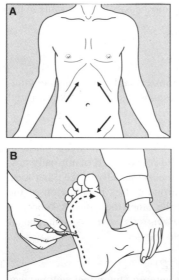

Fig. 27
A. Eliciting abdominal reflex.
B. Eliciting the plantar response.

EXAMINATION OF THE SENSORY SYSTEM

Testing sensation should involve comparison of both sides of the body. It is important to become efficient, as repetition causes loss of the patient's concentration and cooperation.

Anatomy

Localisation of lesions requires an accurate interpretation of the neurological findings and a detailed knowledge of neuroanatomy (Figs 28 and 29).

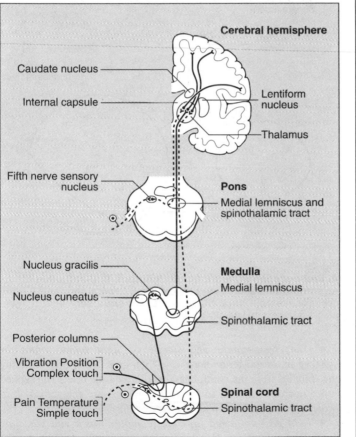

Cerebral hemisphere

Caudate nucleus

Internal capsule

Lentiform nucleus

Thalamus

Fifth nerve sensory nucleus

Pons

Medial lemniscus and spinothalamic tract

Nucleus gracilis

Medulla

Medial lemniscus

Nucleus cuneatus

Spinothalamic tract

Posterior columns

Vibration Position Complex touch

Pain Temperature Simple touch

Spinal cord

Spinothalamic tract

Fig. 28
The main sensory pathways.

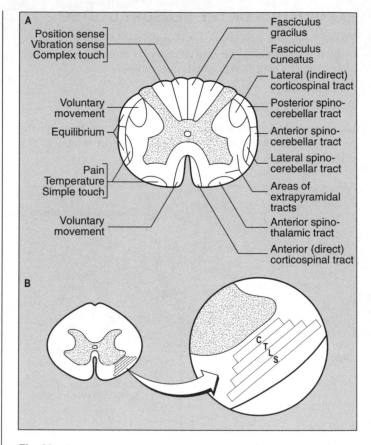

Fig. 29
A. Cross-section of the thoracic spinal cord. B. Distribution of spinothalamic tracts at the cervical level. Cervical segments (C) lie centrally with the thoracic (T), lumbar (L) and sacral segments (S) lying progressively more laterally.

- *Pain*, *temperature* and *simple* or *light touch* sensations synapse in the posterior horns and then cross soon after entering the spinal cord to the contralateral spinothalamic tract. The second order neurones ascend to the thalamus and are relayed as third order neurones to the sensory cortex.

- *Joint position*, *deep pressure*, *complex touch* and *vibration* sensations ascend in the ipsilateral posterior columns to the medulla oblongata. From there, second order neurones cross to reach the thalamus via the medial lemniscus.

Examination sequence

Simple touch

❑ Ask the patient to keep the eyes closed and to report the touch of a point of cotton wool applied at irregular time intervals. Touch, do not stroke, and compare one side with the other.

❑ Map areas of altered sensation on the limbs or trunk by testing from abnormal areas to areas of normal sensation.

Pain

❑ Ask the patient to keep the eyes closed and to distinguish between the blunt and sharp ends of a pin; use a paperclip or a disposable neurotip for this purpose, checking each dermatome as appropriate.

❑ Compare and contrast pain sensation between opposite sides of the body and map areas of altered sensation.

Temperature sensation

❑ Test only to confirm the findings on pinprick when the other sensory modalities are unexpectedly normal (e.g. suspected syringomyelia).

❑ Ask the patient to keep the eyes closed and to distinguish between tubes containing either hot or cold water applied in a random sequence to the skin.

Joint position sense

❑ Hold the patient's terminal phalanx between thumb and forefinger while immobilising the proximal phalanx with the other hand.

❑ Flex and extend the patient's distal interphalangeal joint and ask the patient with the eyes closed to indicate the directions of movement; take care to ensure that the examining fingers do not touch the patient's other digits (Fig. 30).

Vibration sense

❑ Ask the patient to describe the sensations produced by a vibrating 128 cycles/s tuning fork placed on the dorsum of a terminal phalanx (Fig. 31). Ask the patient to report as soon as the vibration stops.

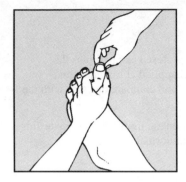

Fig. 30
Testing joint position sense in the great toe.

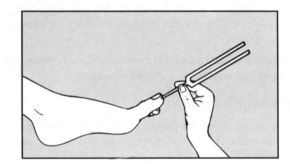

Fig. 31
Testing for vibration sensation.

❑ If vibration sense is impaired, move the tuning fork proximally to establish the level at which it is perceived.

Impairment of joint position and vibration sense usually affects the distal parts of the limbs first. Only if joint position sense is impaired peripherally need similar tests be employed more proximally.

Coordination

The smooth and accurate performance of specific movements requires intact motor, sensory and cerebellar function. Patients vary widely in their ability to coordinate movements and most are less dexterous with the non-dominant hand. Any lesion which causes weakness may be accompanied by clumsiness but incoordination is particularly prominent in the absence of normal sensation (*sensory ataxia*) or in cerebellar dysfunction (*cerebellar ataxia*).

• *Sensory ataxia* is the incoordination resulting from defective proprioception which is normally modified by visual feedback; such patients perform poorly with the eyes closed or in the dark (*rombergism*).

• *Cerebellar ataxia* is an incoordination that is not susceptible to visual compensation; patients tend to 'overshoot' the target even with their eyes open (*dysmetria*), and their movements are clumsy and jerky as the target is approached owing to the intention tremor. Rapid, alternating movements are rendered irregular in force and rhythm (*dysdiadokokinesis*).

Examination sequence

❑ Test rapidly alternating pronation and supination of the forearm by asking the patient to quickly slap the examiner's palm with the front and back of the hand alternately.

❑ Ask the patient to hold the arms outstretched and then to touch the tip of the nose with the tip of each index finger in turn (*finger–nose test*; Fig. 32A).

❑ Ask the patient to place one heel on the opposite knee and then slide the heel down the front of the shin to the ankle and back again. Repeat the test with the other heel (*heel–shin test*; Fig. 32B).

❑ Ask the patient to sit upright without holding on to the arms of the chair and look for signs of truncal ataxia.

❑ Ask the patient to stand unsupported with the feet together and note the degree of sway.

❑ Assess the effect of eye closure on standing balance (*Romberg's test*) and observe the degree of sway when the patient is asked to stand on one leg.

❑ Observe the gait during slow and quick walking and especially as the patient turns. Loss of balance is suggested from the history; difficulty in walking in the dark or with eyes closed suggests sensory ataxia (*rombergism*) but difficulty in walking with the eyes open suggests cerebellar ataxia.

Cortical sensory functions

Lesions of the sensory cortex impair the more discriminative

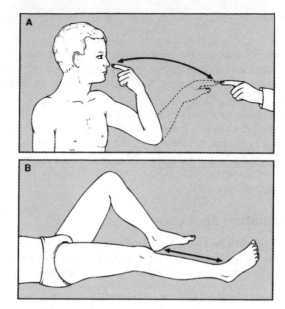

Fig. 32
Tests of limb coordination. A. Finger–nose test. **B.** Heel–shin test.

aspects of sensation. There is no point in testing cortical sensory functions in the presence of a peripheral nerve or cord lesion.

Tests of sensory cortical function

• *Stereognosis* – the ability to distinguish shapes, contours and textures (complex touch).

• *Two-point discrimination* – the ability to perceive two simultaneous stimuli as distinct when separated by minimal distances. Over the fingertips, two points separated by only 2–3 mm can normally be identified, whereas over the leg, the distance may exceed 50 mm. Specially calibrated dividers are available, but an opened-out paperclip makes a convenient and satisfactory 'instrument'.

• *Sensory inattention* – the inability to perceive two simultaneous stimuli at corresponding sites on both sides of the body. A lesion of the parietal cortex is suggested if apparent hemianaesthesia can be demonstrated when two stimuli are applied to both sides simultaneously but not when applied separately to either side.

• *Dyspraxia* – difficulty in the performance of more complex movements may be observed in the absence of incoordination, weakness or sensory defect and suggests cortical dysfunction. Patients with dyspraxia write slowly and with difficulty; the formation of letters may be incomplete and their size variable.

Examination sequence

❏ Ask the patient to perform specific tasks such as dressing or putting on spectacles.

❏ Ask the patient to draw figures such as squares or triangles.

❏ Record a sample of the patient's handwriting to compare with a previous sample.

❏ Randomly apply one or two points of the ends of a paperclip (or pair of dividers) to the skin at varying distances of separation. Ask the patient to keep the eyes closed and to identify whether one or two points can be felt after each stimulus.

❏ Ask the patient to keep the eyes closed and to identify objects such as a key, coin or pen by palpation; take care not to cue the patient with the noise of keys or coins.

❏ Alternatively, ask the patient to identify unseen numbers outlined on the skin.

❏ Demonstrate first that a stimulus is perceived separately on each side then stimulate corresponding areas on each side simultaneously; ask the patient to keep the eyes closed and to report whether sensations are felt on the right side, left side or both sides together. Repeat several times to confirm the finding if sensory inattention is present.

EXAMINATION OF THE CRANIAL NERVES

Olfactory (first cranial) nerve

Loss of the sense of smell (*anosmia*) is much more commonly due to nasal disease than to neurological causes, and enquiry should be made about nasal catarrh. Olfactory nerves are not usually tested unless disorders within the anterior cerebral fossa are suspected, e.g. skull fracture or frontal lobe tumour.

Examination sequence

❑ Test the patency of the nasal airway by asking the patient to sniff.

❑ Test each nostril separately by occluding the other nostril.

❑ Ask the patient to keep the eyes closed and to identify common odours such as an orange or tobacco.

Optic (second cranial) nerve

Examination comprises assessment of visual acuity, visual fields and ophthalmoscopy (p. 119).

Visual acuity
Spectacles should be worn if required, since acuity, not refractive error, is being tested. Near vision can be tested either by asking the patient to read the different typefaces of a newspaper or by using standard reading charts such as the Jaeger card. Distant vision is assessed by reading the standard Snellen types at a distance of 6 metres. The results are recorded as 6/6, 6/18, etc., the latter meaning that at a distance of 6 metres, the patient can just read what should be readable at 18 metres.

Visual fields
Defects in the visual fields resulting from lesions of the visual pathways are shown in Figure 33. The visual fields are assessed clinically by the technique of confrontation (Fig. 34). The test is invalidated if the patient looks away.

Examination sequence
Visual acuity

❑ Ask the patient to wear glasses if appropriate and test each eye separately.

❑ Record the findings for both near and distant vision.

Visual fields

❑ Sit directly opposite the patient and ask the patient to look into the examiner's eyes.

❑ Check first for visual inattention by testing both eyes

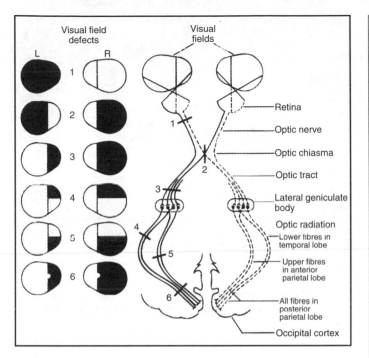

Fig. 33
Visual field defects. 1. Total loss of vision in one eye owing to a lesion of the optic nerve. 2. Bitemporal hemianopia due to compression of the optic chiasma. 3. Right homonymous hemianopia from a lesion of the optic tract. 4. Upper right quadrantic hemianopia from a lesion of the lower fibres of the optic radiation in the temporal lobe. 5. Less commonly a lower quadrantic hemianopia occurs from a lesion of the upper fibres of the optic radiation in the anterior part of the parietal lobe. 6. Right homonymous hemianopia with sparing of the macula from a lesion of the optic radiation in the posterior part of the parietal lobe

simultaneously. With arms outstretched, waggle one or both forefingers and ask the patient to report the side on which movement is observed (Fig. 34A).

❏ Then test each eye separately by asking the patient to cover one eye and to look into the examiner's opposing eye.

❏ Examine the outer aspects of the visual fields by bringing a waggling finger into the field of vision from the periphery at

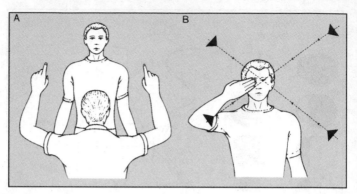

Fig. 34
Testing the visual fields. A. Test for visual inattention with both eyes open. **B.** Test each eye separately with the other eye closed. Approach with a fingertip along the diagonals. Map out any defect carefully.

several points on the circumference of the upper and lower, nasal and temporal quadrants of the visual fields (Fig. 34B).

❏ Ask the patient to state as soon as the movement of the fingertip is observed.

❏ Map out central field defects by moving the fingertip across the visual field.

Oculomotor, trochlear and abducent (third, fourth and sixth cranial) nerves

The sixth cranial nerve supplies the lateral rectus muscle, which moves the eye laterally. The fourth nerve supplies the superior oblique muscle, which is a pure depressor when the eye is adducted. All the other eye movements, including elevation of the upper eyelid, are supplied by the third nerve (Fig. 35). With complete paralysis of the third nerve, the patient cannot open the affected eye. The sympathetic nerve supply to the superior tarsal muscle also raises the upper eyelid slightly and its loss will produce ptosis and miosis – *Horner's syndrome* (Fig. 36).

Inspection of eyes

The pupils are normally round, regular in outline and equal. Their size varies with the intensity of ambient lighting but is usually 3–5 mm in diameter. Constriction of the pupil of less than 3 mm is

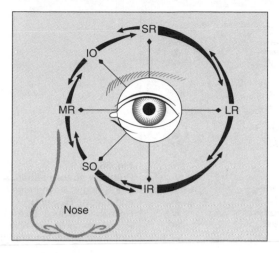

Fig. 35
Testing ocular movements. Medial and lateral rectus (MR – LR) move
the eye medially and laterally respectively. Superior rectus (SR),
assisted by inferior oblique (IO), elevates the eye, and inferior rectus,
assisted by superior oblique (SO), depresses the eye. When the eye is
turned medially, inferior oblique turns the eye upward, superior oblique
moves it downwards. When the eye is turned laterally, superior rectus
elevates it and inferior rectus depresses it.

known as *miosis*, while dilatation above 5 mm in average illumination is called *mydriasis*.

Pupillary reflexes
If a light is shone into one eye, normally both pupils constrict.

- The *direct light reflex* is the reaction of the pupil on the
  stimulated side.
- The *consensual light reflex* is the constriction of the other pupil.
- The *accommodation reflex* is the constriction of the pupils
  occurring in response to convergence of the eyes on a near
  object.

Examination sequence

❑ Note any asymmetry, such as drooping of an eyelid (ptosis) by
  comparing the widths of the palpebral fissures and look for
  asymmetry of pupil diameters.

❑ Using a bright light in a darkened room, approach the eye from

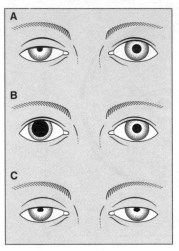

Fig. 36
Pupillary abnormalities. A.
(right) Horner's syndrome (ptosis
and miosis). **B.** (right)
Holmes–Adie pupil. **C.** Argyll
Robertson pupils with bilateral
ptosis and small, irregular pupils.

the side to avoid an accommodation reflex constricting the pupil.
Shine the light into one eye and check that both pupils constrict.

❑ Assess the speed and extent of constriction in each eye
separately, shielding the other from the light while doing so in
order to test both direct and consensual light reflexes.

❑ Ask the patient to gaze into the distance and then to look at a
finger placed near the patient's nose; observe the response of
both pupils.

Impairment or absence of the pupillary reaction to light may be
due to interruption of the afferent or efferent limbs of the reflex
arc. If a pupil constricts only when light is shone into the opposite
eye, i.e. the consensual light reflex is preserved, the efferent pathway
from the midbrain is intact but the patient is blind in that eye. Loss of
the direct light reflex with preservation of the accommodation
reflex, the *Argyll Robertson pupil*, when accompanied by small,
irregular and unequal pupils, suggests neurosyphilis (Fig. 36). The
Holmes–Adie pupil or *myotonic pupil* is a dilated pupil which
reacts sluggishly to both light and accommodation. It is often
unilateral, does not indicate significant neurological disease and is
usually associated with absence of tendon reflexes.

Ocular movements
Disordered movements may result from disorders of the ocular
muscles (ocular myopathies), neuromuscular junction (myasthenia

gravis), ocular nerves or their nuclei, internuclear and supranuclear connections.

Examination sequence

❑ Examine carefully for any squint (*strabismus*).

❑ Ask the patient to fix the gaze on the examining finger and to report if double vision occurs while following the movement of the finger held at a distance of at least 50 cm.

❑ Move the finger up and down, then to the right and up and down, and then to the left and up and down.

❑ Record the directions in which double vision occurs and the images are maximally separated; ask the patient to close one eye at a time to identify which eye is producing the false image.

When double vision (diplopia) develops, the peripheral image is the false image and attributable to the eye whose movement is impaired.

Nystagmus
Nystagmus, involuntary rhythmic oscillations of the eyes, is either pendular or jerking in type.

Examination sequence

❑ Ask the patient to follow a rapidly moving finger in order to accentuate nystagmus.

❑ Record the presence of vertical, horizontal or rotatory nystagmus and the direction of gaze in which nystagmus is most marked.

❑ Note the direction of the fast component of nystagmus, whether it changes direction with the direction of gaze and whether the degree of nystagmus is different in each eye (*ataxic* or *dysconjugate nystagmus*).

○ **Pendular nystagmus** is characterised by oscillations about a central point that are equal in rate and amplitude and may occur in any plane; most commonly it results from a defect in macular vision.

○ **Jerking nystagmus** is characterised by oscillations of the eyes which have both a rapid and a slow component. The direction of the rapid component is conventionally used to define the direction of nystagmus. Thus 'nystagmus to the right' refers to the direction of the rapid component not the direction of gaze in which nystagmus occurs.

Jerking nystagmus may be peripheral or central in origin:

• Peripheral lesions affecting the vestibular apparatus or vestibular nerve produce a unidirectional nystagmus irrespective of the direction of gaze.

• Central lesions in the brain stem or cerebellum produce bidirectional nystagmus (the direction of nystagmus changes with the direction of gaze). Lesions of the medial longitudinal bundle produce bidirectional nystagmus more marked in the abducting eye (dysconjugate or *ataxic nystagmus*)

Trigeminal (fifth cranial) nerve

The trigeminal nerve comprises sensory and motor components; the sensory part supplies sensation to the face, scalp, tongue and buccal mucosa (Fig. 37) and the motor part supplies the muscles of mastication (the pterygoid, masseter and temporalis muscles). In addition, the trigeminal nerve carries the sensory limb of the corneal reflex and both the sensory and motor limbs of the jaw jerk. A pathologically brisk jaw jerk denotes a bilateral upper motor neurone lesion.

Examination sequence

Sensory function

❏ Assess both touch and pain sensation in the territories of the

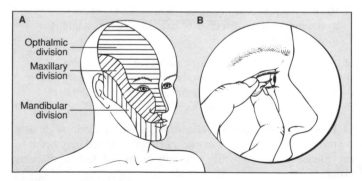

Fig. 37
A. Divisions of the trigeminal nerve. B. Eliciting the corneal reflex.

three sensory divisions (Fig. 37A) using the methods described previously (p. 77).

❑ Compare sensation on both sides of the forehead, cheeks and jaw.

❑ Assess the corneal reflexes by gently touching the edge of the cornea with a wisp of cotton wool, approaching each eye from the side to avoid responses induced by the patient anticipating the stimulus (Fig. 37B). Alternatively, ask the patient to compare the sensation induced by a wisp of cotton wool inserted into each nostril in turn.

Motor function

❑ Ask the patient to open the jaw against resistance; the jaw deviates towards the side of any unilateral weakness of the lateral pterygoid muscles.

❑ Palpate the masseter muscles as the teeth are clenched to assess power and symmetry.

❑ To elicit the jaw jerk, ask the patient to let the mouth hang open, place the examiner's thumb on the chin and strike the thumb with a tendon hammer (Fig. 38).

Facial (seventh cranial) nerve

The motor component of the facial nerve supplies the muscles of facial expression; the sensory component supplies taste sensations from the anterior two-thirds of the tongue via the chorda tympani. Because upper facial movements are innervated from both sides of the motor cortex, unilateral upper motor neurone lesions characteristically reduce movements of the lower part of the face more than the upper part of the face. In contrast, lower motor neurone lesions

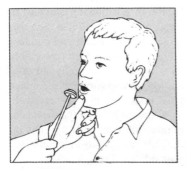

**Fig. 38
Eliciting the jaw jerk.**

affect both upper and lower parts of the face equally. Involuntary facial movements such as blinking, and emotional expressions such as smiling may be preserved or even exaggerated in lesions of the upper motor neurone.

Examination sequence

Motor function

❑ Look for signs of facial paralysis: reduced wrinkling of the forehead, drooping of the corner of the mouth or flattening of the nasolabial fold.

❑ Ask the patient to frown and to look upwards to wrinkle the forehead; ask the patient to shut the eyes as tightly as possible.

❑ Ask the patient to grimace, show the teeth, blow out the cheeks and whistle.

❑ Compare involuntary facial movements by trying to make the patient smile spontaneously.

Sensory function

❑ Test taste (sweet, salt, bitter and sour) using sugar, salt, quinine and vinegar, respectively.

❑ Hold the protracted tongue gently in a swab and use an orange stick to place test substances on each side of the tongue in turn; ask the patient to identify the taste by pointing to the word 'sweet', 'salt', 'bitter' or 'sour' written on cards.

Vestibulocochlear (eighth cranial) nerve

The eighth cranial nerve comprises two distinct components: vestibular and auditory. Though vestibular function cannot be fully evaluated at the bedside, the induction of positional nystagmus in response to sudden changes in head position (*Hallpike manoeuvres*) suggests a labyrinthine disorder. Sensorineural and conduction deafness can be distinguished using a tuning fork (preferably 256 cycles/s, though 128 cycles/s will serve). Normally, air conduction is better than bone conduction. In auditory nerve damage (*sensorineural deafness*) the normal relationship is preserved. In *conduction deafness* due to wax or a foreign body in the meatus or disease of the middle ear, bone conduction may be better than air conduction because masking of the external sounds in the affected ear results in 'better' hearing on that side.

Examination sequence

❏ Test the hearing of each ear in turn by asking the patient to repeat numbers or words whispered into the ear while occluding the meatus of the opposite ear using finger pressure.

❏ Place the base of the vibrating tuning fork on the mastoid bone until the sound fades. Then place the tip of the tuning fork over the meatus. Normally the sound should become audible (*Rinne's test*).

❏ Place the base of the vibrating tuning fork on the vertex of the skull and ask the patient whether the sound is midline or heard preferentially in one ear (*Weber's test*).

❏ Inspect the external ear passages and tympanic membranes using an auriscope if hearing is impaired or if earache is a problem (p. 117).

Glossopharyngeal (ninth cranial) nerve

Most of the motor functions of the glossopharyngeal nerve are closely associated with the function of the tenth cranial nerve; sensory functions include taste sensation to the posterior third of the tongue and pharyngeal sensation. Testing the sensation of the posterior tongue and pharynx is unpleasant for the patient and should only be performed when it is important to define ninth nerve function precisely.

Examination sequence

❏ Test taste by applying the test substance with the point of an orange stick as described previously (p. 92).

❏ Touch the posterior pharyngeal wall to evoke the gag reflex, whose sensory limb is the glossopharyngeal nerve and motor limb, the vagus nerve.

Vagus (tenth cranial) nerve

The vagus nerve supplies the muscles of the vocal cords and soft palate. Lesions of the vagus nerve or its recurrent laryngeal branch may give rise to dysphonia, a '*bovine*' cough and a nasal quality to the voice. In bilateral lesions, the soft palate fails to elevate; unilateral lesions produce failure to elevate the affected side of the soft palate resulting in the uvula and posterior pharyngeal wall deviating laterally towards the unaffected side.

Examination sequence

❑ Ask the patient to cough and to vocalise the vowel sounds, 'a', 'e', 'i', 'o', 'u'.

❑ Observe the movements of the soft palate, uvula and posterior pharynx as the patient utters a prolonged 'ah', or while testing the gag reflex.

Spinal accessory (eleventh cranial) nerve

This supplies the sternomastoid and upper trapezius muscles. The sternomastoid turns the head to the opposite side and the trapezius raises the shoulders. A weak trapezius often produces apparent asymmetry of arm lengths.

Examination sequence

❑ Examine the bulk and power of the sternomastoid and trapezius muscles.

❑ Look from behind the patient for signs of muscle wasting of trapezius and note the resting position of the hands along the trunk.

❑ Ask the patient to shrug both shoulders against resistance.

❑ Test both sternomastoids together by asking the patient to flex the neck by pressing the chin downwards against the examiner's hand.

❑ Test each sternomastoid separately by asking the patient to rotate the chin to each side in turn against resistance.

Hypoglossal (twelfth cranial) nerve

Lower motor neurone lesions of the hypoglossal nerve produce wasting and fasciculation of the tongue; unilateral paralysis causes deviation of the tongue towards the paralysed side.

Examination sequence

❑ Inspect the tongue in the floor of the mouth for evidence of wasting and fasciculation.

❑ Ask the patient to protrude the tongue and look for deviation to one side; then ask the patient to press the tongue against each cheek while applying resistance.

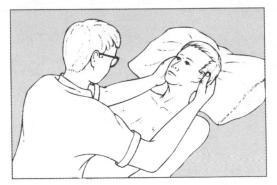

Fig. 39
Testing for meningeal irritation (neck stiffness).

Supplementary tests

Meningeal irritation

Inflammation of the meninges due to infection or blood in the sub-arachnoid space evokes reflex spasm in the paravertebral muscles. In the cervical region this causes painful restriction of passive flexion of the neck (*neck stiffness*). In the early stages of meningeal irritation, spasm may be more easily demonstrable if the neck is flexed abruptly (Fig. 39). Meningeal irritation also restricts passive hip flexion, inducing spasm of the hamstrings that prevents full extension of the knee (Kernig's sign).

Nerve root irritation

When lumbar nerve roots are compressed, e.g. prolapsed interver-tebral disc, stretching of the affected nerve may give rise to pain in the lower back or buttock. The sciatic nerve roots are tested by straight leg raising (Fig. 40). Normally, 90 degrees of pain-free hip flexion should be possible. Femoral nerve root compression causes limitation of hip extension.

Examination sequence

Meningeal irritation

❏ Ask the patient to flex the neck to make the chin touch the chest.

❏ Alternatively, place both hands beneath the patient's occiput then slowly flex the neck.

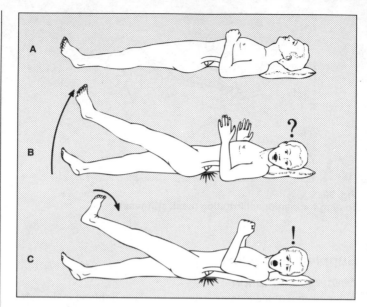

Fig. 40
Straight leg raising. A. Patient lying supine is free from pain.
B. Straight leg raising is limited by tension of the root over the
prolapsed disc causing pain. **C.** Tension and pain are increased by
dorsiflexion of the foot.

❑ Look for Kernig's sign by positioning the patient supine with
one leg extended. Then flex the other knee and hip to 90 degrees
and then extend the knee, keeping the hip flexed.

Nerve root irritation

❑ To test the sciatic nerve roots, position the patient supine and
slowly flex the hip with the knee fully extended to stretch the
nerve roots.

❑ Ask the patient to report any pain as soon as it is experienced
and to indicate the site of the pain.

❑ Look for tenderness of the sciatic nerve by compressing the
greater sciatic notch.

❑ To test the femoral nerve roots, position the patient prone and
slowly extend the hip with the knee flexed to 90 degrees. Ask
the patient to report any pain as soon as it is experienced.

The unconscious patient

Patients in coma do not respond to pain or verbal commands appropriately. It is important when possible, to obtain an account of the events leading up to clouding of consciousness from relatives, friends, neighbours or passers-by. The history of previous medical conditions may also provide important information relevant to the development of coma. When assessing an unconscious patient, the priority is to exclude factors that may be contributing to cerebral hypoxaemia or exacerbating cerebral damage, e.g. airway obstruction, anaemia, cardiac or respiratory failure, hypotension, hypertension, hypoglycaemia, drug or alcohol intoxication, meningitis and systemic infections. Only thereafter should the examination proceed to assessing the cause of the unconsciousness and finally its severity. The severity of the coma and its prognosis can be assessed using the 'Glasgow Coma Scale' to measure motor, ocular and verbal responses to a variety of stimuli.

DIAGNOSTIC PROCESS

It is important to remember the principal signs attributable to lesions of different components of the nervous system. They may not, however, all be present in every situation.

Features of upper motor neurone (pyramidal tract) lesions

- Paresis or paralysis
- Hypertonia of spastic type
- Increased tendon reflexes and clonus
- Absence of cutaneous reflexes
- An extensor plantar response

Features of lower motor neurone lesions

- Paresis or paralysis
- Hypotonia
- Muscle wasting
- Muscle fasciculation
- Diminished or absent tendon reflexes

Features of cerebellar lesions

- Limb ataxia
- Truncal ataxia
- Intention tremor

- Jerking nystagmus (bidirectional)
- Scanning dysarthria

Features of mixed sensorimotor polyneuropathies

- Impaired sensation affecting all modalities
- Sensory loss occurring in a 'stocking' ± 'glove' distribution
- Muscle wasting and fasciculation particularly in the distal limbs
- Muscle weakness particularly of distal limb movements
- Diminished or absent tendon reflexes

Features of posterior column lesions (ipsilateral)

- Sensory ataxia of the limbs
- Preservation of pain and temperature sensations
- Impaired joint position sense
- Impaired vibration sense
- Preservation of the tendon reflexes

Features of spinothalamic tract lesions (contralateral)

- Dissociate sensory loss:
  - impairment of pain and temperature sensation
  - preservation of vibration, touch and joint position sense
- Loss of tendon reflexes
- Preservation of motor function

Features of extrinsic spinal cord lesions

- Early radicular pain and localised spinal tenderness
- Preservation of perineal sensation (sacral sparing)
- Loss of sensation over many dermatomes
- Progression to sphincter disturbance
- Spastic paresis or paralysis

Features of intrinsic spinal cord lesions

- Late development of pain or spinal tenderness
- Loss of perineal sensation (saddle anaesthesia)
- Dissociate sensory loss (selective loss of pain sensation)
- Early onset of sphincter dysfunction
- Spastic paresis or paralysis

Neurological patterns of disease

The identification of damaged neural structures is followed by the definition of the site or sites of their involvement:

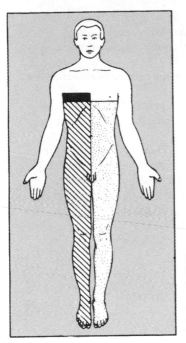

Fig. 41
Hemisection of the spinal cord (Brown–Sequard syndrome).
Ipsilateral loss of joint position sense (hatched area); contralateral loss of pain and temperature sense (dotted area).

- Single lesion, e.g. hemisection of the spinal cord, may affect diverse functions (Fig. 41)
- Multiple lesions, e.g. optic neuropathy associated with spinal cord signs in multiple sclerosis
- Systematised lesions with similar types of neural fibres affected throughout the nervous system, e.g. motor neurone disease with loss of upper motor and lower motor neurones
- Generalised disorders of the central nervous system, e.g. multi-infarct dementia and chronic CNS infection.

Summary points

✦ The history suggests the nature of the pathological process; the examination indicates its extent.
✦ Standing patients who lose consciousness may not remember falling. Eye witness account may be very helpful.
✦ Examination of the mental state and cognitive function helps avoid missing the diagnoses of dementia and/or psychotic disorder.

+ Symptoms usually antedate signs; apparent signs without corresponding symptoms are usually spurious.
+ Ask the patient to report any double vision when testing eye movements.
+ Compare like with like during the neurological examination of the limbs.
+ Reflexes may be absent or exaggerated in healthy people.
+ Plantar responses can be difficult either to elicit or interpret if the feet are cold.
+ Perform the plantar response slowly while applying firm pressure; stop with the first obvious movement of the big toe.
+ Prolongation of the sensory examination can produce inconsistent findings due to patient fatigue; examination may need to be piecemeal in frail or ill patients.

The locomotor system 6

HISTORY

Cardinal symptoms

- Pain
- Joint stiffness
- Joint swelling
- Immobility

○ **Pain** should be assessed as described previously (p. 5). The pattern of pain in relation to rest and physical activity is often characteristic. In inflammatory joint disorders such as rheumatoid arthritis, both pain and stiffness are worse after resting and gradually improve as the joints are used. In degenerative joint disorders such as osteoarthrosis, joints are more comfortable at rest and exercise exacerbates joint pains.

○ **Joint stiffness** is common to both inflammatory and degenerative arthritides. In rheumatoid arthritis, stiffness typically exhibits diurnal variation with '*immobility stiffness*' lasting an hour or longer after rising from bed in the morning and with stiffness and pain recurring at the end of the day.

○ **Joint swelling** is common following trauma. In the absence of trauma, swelling suggests inflammation. The absence of swelling in painful joints (*arthralgia*) can be a useful pointer to some disorders such as viral infections and polymyalgia rheumatica.

○ **Immobility** may be the result of a number of factors including joint pain, stiffness or muscle wasting due to physical inactivity. Often a combination of these factors is involved. Occasionally, an abnormal degree of mobility will be apparent either as a result of the loss of supporting tendons or owing to abnormal tissue laxity as in the *hypermobility syndrome*.

General considerations

The locomotor system includes the joints, the muscles and the tendons which move the joints, and the bones and ligaments which provide support. Though any of these components can be affected by disease, joints are the most commonly disordered. All are frequently involved in injury, but sometimes patients incorrectly attribute their problem to minor injury in the absence of another explanation. The degree of functional disability is important to establish so that illness can be seen in the context of the activities of daily living (ADL; p. 6).

Patterns of joint involvement

Special note should be made of the pattern and symmetry of joint involvement, the sequence of involvement and whether symptoms moved from one joint to another (*flitting arthritis*), or progressed to affect an increasing number of joints (*additive arthritis*). In inflammatory joint disorders, other connective tissues including blood vessels, skin, muscle, tendons and fascia may also be involved.

PHYSICAL EXAMINATION

The locomotor system is examined by inspection and palpation both at rest and during movement. The examination may be performed in part or as a whole (Fig. 42). Nearly all the structures are paired, facilitating comparison of the affected part with its normal counterpart. Abnormalities such as the restriction of joint movement, joint swelling, muscle wasting and injuries can be measured and/or recorded using diagrams.

○ **Posture and gait** alter with age and disease particularly of the spine, e.g. kyphosis and kyphoscoliosis (p. 36). Thoracic kyphosis (increased anteroposterior curvature of the spine) is a common abnormality in the elderly resulting from spinal osteoporosis (deficiency of bone matrix) or, less commonly, osteomalacia (demineralisation of bone). The rhythm of the gait is often disturbed by pain. The patient takes the weight off the painful leg as quickly as possible and the timing is *dot–dash, dot–dash,* painful–normal, painful–normal. Painless loss or impairment of joint movement as from bony or fibrous fusion, causes a contrary pattern of gait, in that the long pause is on the abnormal leg, i.e. *dash–dot, dash–dot,* abnormal–normal, abnormal–normal. A *waddling gait* is the result of gluteal muscle dysfunction as is typically present in bilateral congenital dislocation of the hips. Characteristic gaits of neurological origin include the spastic gait of hemiplegia, the ataxic gait of cerebellar disease, the festinant, shuffling gait of parkinsonism and the high-stepping gait of foot drop.

○ **Joints, muscles and related structures.** Examination of the appropriate structure is much easier if the examiner demonstrates which movement the patient is being asked to perform. At the same time, the normal range of movement will be apparent for the purpose of comparison.

○ **Passive movement and palpation.** When active movement of a joint is impaired, or if abnormal mobility is suspected, the cause may become apparent during passive movements.

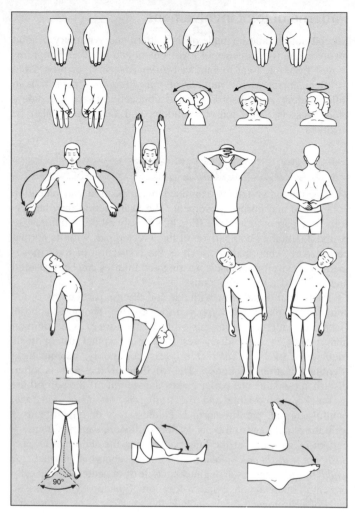

Fig. 42
Examination of active movements.

Examination sequence

General observations

❑ Observe any abnormality of the posture or gait.

❑ Inspect the joints, muscles and related structures.

- ❑ Compare the affected joint with that of the other limb to detect less obvious differences.

- ❑ Compare the temperature of any swollen joint with that of the same joint on the opposite side.

- ❑ Assess the bulk and strength of the adjacent muscles.

- ❑ Determine if any muscle wasting is due to joint immobility, physical inactivity or primary neuromuscular disorder.

Active movements

- ❑ Check active before passive joint movements particularly if pain is present.

- ❑ Measure the range of active movements.

Passive movements

- ❑ Passive movements need not be tested if active movement is unimpaired, unless an abnormal degree of mobility is being sought.

- ❑ Observe the patient's face during joint movement looking for any indication of pain.

- ❑ Palpate for coarse crepitus; if the articular cartilage is severely damaged it may be audible.

- ❑ Localise any points of tenderness and try to identify the tissue involved by stressing the affected structure. (Ligamentous lesions cause pain during both passive and active movement; muscle lesions cause pain during active contraction even without movement and tendon rupture causes loss of all active movements with normal passive movement.)

Examination of specific joints

- ❑ Inspect the dorsum of the hands and wrists; ask the patient to clench the fists, show the palms, touch the little finger with the thumb and put the wrists through a full range of movements.

- ❑ Inspect the elbows and ask the patient to bend, then straighten the elbows fully.

- ❑ Test abduction and external and internal rotation of the shoulder by asking the patient to raise the arms above the head, then touch the back of the neck and then the small of the back.

❏ Ask the patient to fully extend and flex the neck, and then to try to touch the tip of each shoulder with the ear, to test lateral flexion, and with the chin to test rotation.

❏ Test spinal flexion and extension by asking the patient to attempt to touch the toes with the knees straight and to lean backwards; use a tape measure to assess the maximal spinal flexion and extension at the level of the posterior iliac spines (*Schober's test*).

❏ Test lateral flexion of the spine by asking the patient to slide the hand as far as possible down the lateral side of each thigh, and rotation by turning head and shoulders to the right and left.

❏ Test the sacroiliac joints with the patient in the left lateral position; compress the bony pelvis by leaning firmly on the anterior iliac crest. Alternatively, stress the sacroiliac joints by passive flexion of one hip while maintaining hyperextension of the other hip. Both manoeuvres provoke pain locally if there is active sacroiliitis.

❏ Measure hip rotation by attempting to put the extended lower limb through a 90 degree arc; use the position of the patient's foot as an indicator when assessing the range of movements in flexion, extension, abduction and adduction.

❏ Inspect the knee joint; ask the patient to move the joint from full extension to full flexion.

❏ Check the integrity of the cruciate ligaments by assessing the

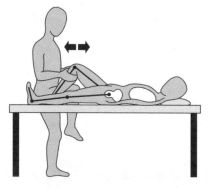

Fig. 43
Assessing the cruciate ligaments of the knee joint.

degree of anteroposterior movement of the knee joint; with the knee in the semi-flexed position, rock the tibia backwards and forwards while immobilising the foot by sitting on it (Fig. 43).

❑ Check the integrity of the collateral ligaments by assessing the degree of lateral movement of the knee joint with the leg straight (Fig. 44).

❑ To test for a knee joint effusion, 'massage' first the medial side of the joint with one hand and then the lateral side of the joint. Observe any filling of the anteromedial aspect indicating an effusion. Where there is a visible swelling, gently compress any fluid from the suprapatellar pouch with one hand and with the other hand, depress the patella abruptly down onto the femur (Fig. 45). A distinct '*tap*' indicates the presence of fluid rather than synovial thickening.

❑ Inspect the ankle joint; ask the patient to flex and extend the ankle joint.

❑ To assess the subtalar joint, ask the patient to invert and evert the foot.

❑ Inspect the feet for any abnormality, e.g. flattening of the arches, callosities or deformities.

Summary points

✦ The pattern of joint pain and stiffness distinguishes inflammatory from degenerative disorders.

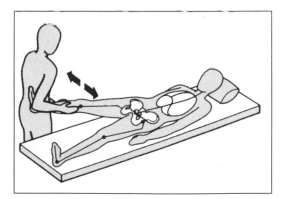

Fig. 44
Assessing the collateral ligaments of the knee joint.

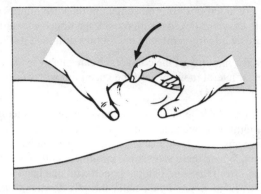

Fig. 45
Testing for knee joint effusions by the patellar tap.

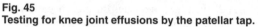

✦ The posture and gait may help characterise osteogenic, arthrogenic and neurogenic disorders.
✦ In painful joints, examine active movements before passive movements.
✦ Inflammation is suggested by the presence of pain, redness, heat and impaired function.
✦ Joint deformity is an unreliable guide to the degree of functional disability.

General examination 7

Those aspects of examination which do not readily fit into any one system are now described and include:

- General observations
- The hands
- The skin
- The head and face
- The eyes, including ophthalmoscopy
- The ears, including auriscopy
- Examination of swellings
- Examination of the neck
- Examination of the breasts

GENERAL OBSERVATIONS

Evidence elicited in the course of the general examination is often highly significant. It may be available to the alert clinician from the moment of first seeing the patient, even before taking the history. Junior students should make a conscious effort to acquire this skill by observing patients carefully.

Demeanour

The patient's demeanour and mood will be readily apparent from careful observation and analysis of the patient's posture, gait, dress and behaviour. Both the verbal and non-verbal communication ('body language') give important and often complementary information.

Abnormal colour

The normal colour of the face depends largely upon variations in skin blood flow and the amounts of melanin and haemoglobin present.

○ **Anaemia** is often best appreciated by examining the conjunctivae and buccal mucosa and by comparing nail-bed and skin-crease colour with that of the examiner.

○ **Cyanosis** appears as a purplish tinge and is attributable to excessive concentrations of reduced haemoglobin.

- *Peripheral cyanosis* occurs with excessive extraction of oxygen from the capillaries owing to low rates of blood flow; in a temperate climate, the affected extremities are cold and blue.

- *Central cyanosis* is more obvious in the tongue and lips than the nail-beds. It occurs when the concentration of desaturated haemoglobin in the arterial blood is at least 40 g per litre. It follows that it cannot be present in a patient who is both hypoxic and severely anaemic. Central cyanosis is best distinguished from peripheral cyanosis by the presence of warm though blue extremities; however, both may coexist, e.g. in a patient with cardiac failure with pulmonary oedema. Central cyanosis is commonly due to respiratory failure but also occurs in polycythaemia, veno-arterial pulmonary shunts or abnormal forms of haemoglobin such as methaemoglobin and sulphaemoglobin.

○ **Melanin.** Increased skin pigmentation due to melanin results from sunlight, chronic inflammation, deposition of heavy metals or over-production of melanocyte-stimulating hormone as in Addison's disease. Reduction in melanin results from lack of sunlight, hypopituitarism, vitiligo, albinism and phenylketonuria.

○ **Bilirubin.** Jaundice is usually seen in the sclera and beneath the tongue before it is obvious in the skin. It may be missed if the patient is examined in artificial light.

Abnormal movements

Involuntary movements such as choreoathetosis, tremors and tics due to disorders of the central nervous system are described on page 69.

Abnormal sounds

A hoarse, gruff voice is characteristic in severe hypothyroidism and is caused by myxoedematous thickening of the vocal cords. A nasal quality of speech indicates a cleft palate or paralysis of the soft palate. Hoarseness, loss of singing voice and difficulty in phonating vowel sounds ('a, e, i, o, u') suggest vocal cord paralysis due to recurrent laryngeal nerve palsy. *Stridor,* an inspiratory, crowing sound, indicates obstruction of the larynx, trachea or major bronchi.

Abnormal odours

Halitosis, a malodorous breath, suggests poor dental hygiene, gingivitis or bronchiectasis. Foul-smelling, faeculent belching is characteristic of a gastrocolic fistula. The sweet smell of acetone in the breath is typical of severe diabetic ketoacidosis; though obvious to some individuals, others may be unable to detect it. A characteristic, sickly smell to the breath, *fetor hepaticus*, occurs in hepatic failure. The smell of marijuana or alcohol should prompt enquiries about a patient's drug and alcohol usage.

Nutritional status

In adults this is best assessed in terms of *body mass index* (BMI) – weight (kg)/height (m)^2.

	BMI
Underweight	<18
Normal	18–25
Overweight	26–29
Obese	30–39
Morbid obesity	40+

Hydration

Salt and water depletion are common in patients with vomiting, diarrhoea, excessive sweating or polyuria. The skin becomes dry, lax and inelastic (*loss of tissue turgor*) and the blood pressure falls. However, a dry tongue may be the result of mouth-breathing and is an unreliable sign of water depletion and often misleading.

Generalised oedema results from either fluid overload, e.g. cardiac failure, or hypoproteinaemia, e.g. nephrotic syndrome, malnutrition or malabsorption. Fluid overload can be distinguished from hypoproteinaemia by the presence of an elevated JVP. In the ambulant patient, pitting oedema can first be detected at the ankles by firm pressure applied for at least 5 seconds. In patients confined to bed, oedema is often marked over the sacrum.

Body temperature

The normal body temperature as measured in the axilla ranges from 36.5–37.0°C. The rectal temperature is about 0.5°C higher. In accidental hypothermia, a special low-reading thermometer should be used.

Examination sequence

General observations

❑ Observe the patient's posture, dress and behaviour while the history is being recorded.

- Observe non-verbal communication (eye-to-eye contact, facial expressions, 'body language').

- Measure the patient's weight and height, calculate the body mass index (BMI).

- Assess the state of hydration carefully in patients with suspected salt and water depletion.

- Look for loss of skin turgor.

- Look for oedema in the dependent areas including the ankles if mobile and the sacrum. Where present, determine its extent.

- Check the patient's temperature if appropriate.

HANDS

After the initial general appraisal of the patient, the specific physical examination often begins with inspection of the hands. Many people express themselves gesticulating with their hands; indeed, the dumb communicate through their hands. Much can be learned about the patient from the appearance of the nails, e.g. well-groomed, bitten, ingrained with dirt or stained with tobacco. Innumerable observations of diagnostic value can be made in this way and include:

- **Skin:** spider telangiectases in cirrhosis of the liver (p. 115)
- **Subcutaneous tissue:** tender areas in the finger pulps in infective endocarditis (*Osler's nodes*)
- **Nails:** *splinter haemorrhages* in infective endocarditis; flattening or 'spooning' (*koilonychia*) in iron deficiency; pitting in psoriasis
- **Muscles:** diffuse wasting and fasciculation in motor neurone disease
- **Tendons:** xanthomatous nodules in hypercholesterolaemia
- **Joints:** spindling of proximal interphalangeal joints in rheumatoid arthritis
- **Bones:** osteophytes of terminal interphalangeal joints (*Heberden's nodes*) in osteoarthrosis.

On palpation, the hot moist palm of hyperthyroidism contrasts with the cold, rough skin of myxoedema. *Finger clubbing* refers to a bulbous swelling of the terminal phalanges of the fingers and toes. Clubbing is occasionally congenital but its development usually indicates serious disease of the lungs or heart, and sometimes of the gut or liver. It is best confirmed by the presence of excess

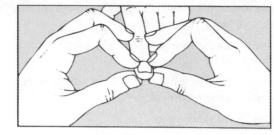

Fig. 46
Testing nail bed fluctuation in finger clubbing.

nail-bed fluctuation together with increased convexity of the nail and loss of the hyponychial angle at the base of the nail.

Examination for finger clubbing

❑ Inspect the digit to assess the nail-bed angle.

❑ Rest the finger to be examined on the pulp of the examiner's thumbs; palpate the base of the nail bed with both forefingers, pressing first with one finger and then the other. Fluctuation gives a floating sensation between the fingers (Fig. 46).

EXAMINATION OF THE SKIN

Examination of the skin and adnexae is normally integrated into the general examination. If the patient's problem is primarily dermatological, the skin should be examined in its entirety. This consists largely of inspection supplemented by palpation to assess the texture of the skin, the consistency of a lesion and the local temperature.

History

Points of special importance should include contact with infectious fevers, scabies or sexually transmitted disease. The purchase of new clothing or jewellery, the application of a new cosmetic or hair dye or recent contact with plants may be the cause of a skin eruption. Systemic or local use of medicaments, with or without medical advice, may be responsible for an immediate or delayed hypersensitivity reaction (urticaria or dermatitis). Some skin lesions are manifestations of systemic disorders, for example erythema nodosum.

Dermatological glossary

○ **A macule** is a small circumscribed discoloration of the skin, such as a freckle.

○ **A papule** is a palpable lesion raised above the surrounding surface of the skin.

○ **A vesicle** (*blister*) is a lesion consisting of liquid within the epidermis or dermis.

○ **A bulla** is a larger variety of vesicle.

○ **A pustule** is a purulent vesicle.

○ **Erythema**, reddening of the skin, is a component of many skin rashes.

○ **Urticaria**, raised pale areas of skin due to interstitial fluid surrounded by erythema, is an allergic response characterised by capillary dilatation induced by an axon reflex.

○ **Eczema**, an eruption characterised by scaling or desquamation due to abnormal maturation of the skin, is associated with allergic disorders in atopic subjects.

Common dermatological lesions

○ **Hirsutism** in females (excessive facial and body hair) is a common finding; on rare occasions it is associated with an endocrinopathy such as the polycystic ovaries syndrome.

○ **Loss of axillary and pubic hair** suggests hypopituitarism or chronic liver failure.

○ **Purpura** is spontaneous bleeding into the skin, which varies in appearance from large areas of bruising (*ecchymoses*) to the smallest lesions (*petechiae*). It occurs in response to increased capillary fragility or from thrombocytopenia. Petechial haemorrhages, often the first manifestation of an acquired haemorrhagic disorder, may be detected only in the legs because of the increased hydrostatic pressure in the ambulant patient.

○ **Spider naevi** are telangiectases with a central arterial dot from which radiate several dilated vessels, all of which can be obliterated by central pressure. They occur in health and in pregnancy but the presence of five or more spider naevi suggests cirrhosis of the liver.

○ **Campbell de Morgan spots** consist of small bright red or bluish *haemangiomas*, especially on the trunk. They are present in many elderly patients and are of no clinical significance. They can be made paler by firm pressure conveniently applied by a pin head but unlike telangiectases, cannot easily be made to disappear.

○ **Seborrhoeic keratosis** usually appears as small, fleshy, yellow-brown papules on the trunk due to basal cell papillomas and are unrelated to the sebaceous glands. Their numbers increase markedly with age and are of no clinical significance. They are also common in immunocompromised disorders, e.g. HIV-related disease.

○ **Puncture marks** suggest the possibilities of drug abuse and infections such as hepatitis B and HIV.

○ **Cutaneous striae** are linear markings sometimes seen on the breasts, thighs and abdomen; those of recent origin are pink while older striae are whitish. They are due to stretching of the skin associated with rapid weight gain due to obesity, ascites or pregnancy. In Cushing's disease or as a result of high-dosage adrenocorticosteroid treatment, purple striae appear over the pectoral regions and upper arms, the lower abdomen and upper thighs.

○ **Erythema nodosum**, characterised by painful, reddish-brown lumps on the shins, is an allergic reaction to various drugs, allergens or infections including sarcoidosis and primary tuberculosis.

○ **Skin tumours** may be benign or malignant, primary or secondary. Basal cell carcinomas (rodent ulcers) are the commonest skin cancers and are often found on the face in the elderly. They rarely metastasise though are locally invasive. In contrast, squamous cell carcinoma (*epithelioma*) is a rapidly growing tumour which may spread to adjacent tissues and the lymph nodes at an early stage. *Melanomas* (*melanocytic naevi*) are benign moles; malignant transformation is rare but is suggested by enlargement, local itch, ulceration, colour change or the development of metastases.

Examination sequence

❑ Inspect the entire surface area of the patient, especially the scalp, umbilicus, natal cleft, perineum and skin flexures.

❑ Describe in detail any lesions found.

HEAD AND FACE

Attention has already been drawn to the transient facial expressions which convey important non-verbal information about the patient. The patient's facial appearance may also be pathognomonic of specific disorders. For example, the asymmetry of a lower motor neurone facial nerve palsy, the immobile stare of parkinsonism, the startled appearance of hyperthyroidism or the epicanthic folds in Down's syndrome. Other features may suggest underlying disease. For example, bilateral parotid gland swelling may occur in alcoholic liver disease or sarcoidosis.

Mouth

Routine examination of the mouth comprises inspection of the lips, tongue, teeth, gums, tonsils, palate, mucosa of the cheeks, floor of the mouth and the oropharynx. The colour of the mucosa gives a useful diagnostic clue to anaemia. Carcinoma should be considered in the differential diagnosis of any chronic ulcer in or around the mouth. A characteristic feature is the hardness of the edge of an ulcer, best assessed by palpation with a gloved finger. A biopsy is essential when suspicion is aroused.

○ **The tongue.** Cyanosis of the tongue is a good guide to central cyanosis (p. 110). Diffuse atrophy of the filiform papillae results in the smooth clean-looking tongue of iron or vitamin B_{12} deficiency. Excessive furring, by contrast, is of little diagnostic significance in spite of the concern it may cause.

○ **The teeth** are commonly affected by caries and they often become loose as the result of periodontitis and recession of the gums due to chronic gingivitis. These disorders may not only produce local symptoms but are also important portals of entry for organisms causing infective endocarditis.

○ **The tonsils** enlarge to reach a maximum between the ages of 8 and 12 years, after which involution usually takes place.

○ **The oropharynx.** Pus from infection in the nose may sometimes be visible tracking down the back of the throat.

Examination sequence

❑ Ask the patient to open the mouth widely.

❑ Examine the mouth, tongue, teeth and tonsils carefully using a spatula and pen torch.

❑ Examine the oropharynx by depressing the tongue with a spatula and asking the patient to say 'Ah' thereby elevating the soft palate.

Ears

Inspection of the pinna of the ears may reveal tophi diagnostic of gout. Testing the hearing is described on page 93. Auriscopic

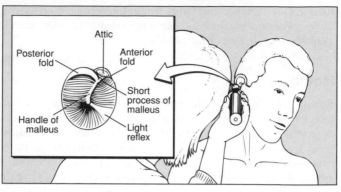

Fig. 47
Auriscopic examination.

examination is indicated if there is earache or deafness. The normal drum is pearly grey, and a cone of reflected light is seen radiating at about 5 o'clock from the centre (Fig. 47). In acute otitis media, the drum may be red, bulging and without a light reflex.

Examination sequence

❏ Inspect the external ear for abnormalities.

❏ Gently retract the pinna of the ear upwards and backwards to straighten the external meatus and facilitate the insertion of the spectrum of the auriscope (Fig. 47).

❏ Identify and examine the tympanic membranes.

Eyes

There may be obvious abnormalities seen from a distance such as puffiness of the face and eyelids in myxoedema and the proptosis and lid retraction in hyperthyroidism. Ptosis may affect one or both eyes, e.g. a partial unilateral ptosis and a small pupil suggests a lesion of the cervical sympathetic nerves (Horner's syndrome). Closer inspection is required to examine the eyelids, the ocular and palpebral conjunctiva (useful sites for checking clinical evidence of jaundice and anaemia), the iris and the pupil. Bluish discoloration of the sclerae is typical of severe, chronic iron deficiency and *osteogenesis imperfecta*.

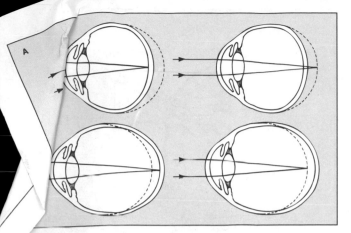

...thalmoscopy. **A.** Hypermetropic (long-sighted) eye. **B.** Myopic (short-sighted) eye.

OPHTHALMOSCOPY

Inspection of the fundi is an important component of the clinical examination. In different subjects, the colour and the form of the visible structures will be seen to be as variable as the facies. Familiarity with the range of normal appearances is therefore essential. Students are strongly advised to buy an ophthalmoscope. Select a model which has an interchangeable auriscope and learn to use several different models before buying the model that suits best.

○ **The ophthalmoscope** contains a wheel carrying up to 30 lenses, arranged according to their focal length, which may be rotated in turn behind the hole in the mirror. The number of each lens corresponds to its focal length expressed in dioptres. A dioptre is the reciprocal of the focal length in metres; for example 2 dioptres corresponds to a focal length of half a metre.

○ **Convex (+)** lenses bring the focal point nearer so that anterior parts of the eye can be examined. They are essential for obtaining a clear view of the fundus after removal of the lens of the eye for cataract or if the patient or the clinician is significantly hypermetropic (Fig. 48A).

○ **Concave (–)** lenses will be required if either the patient or clinician is significantly myopic (Fig. 48B).

Although many lesions can be seen through the untreated pupil,

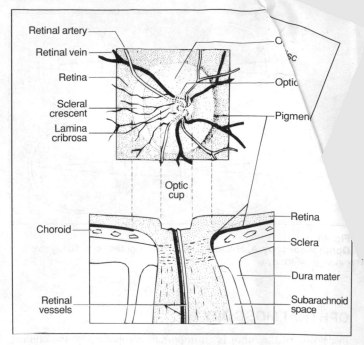

Fig. 49
Normal right optic disc.

for a thorough examination, the pupils may need to be dilated; however, mydriatics should be avoided in patients with acute (closed angle) glaucoma. When viewing the normal fundus from a distance, reflection of the ophthalmoscope light by the retina produces a '*red reflex*'. If a dense cataract is present, the red reflex is lost and the pupil will appear greyish-white owing to the reflecting effect of the cataract itself. Lesser degrees of opacity absorb the light and so appear black. The macula is situated about two discs' width to the temporal side of the lower pole of the optic disc. It appears as a small, dull red patch, darker than the remainder of the fundus. In the centre there is often a little glistening white dot which is due to reflection of light from the fovea. Lesions in this area tend to cause serious loss of vision. The appearance of a normal (right) optic disc is shown in Figure 49.

Indications for ophthalmoscopy

Ophthalmoscopy is indicated in patients with visual symptoms or

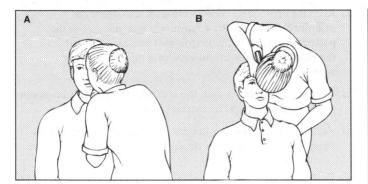

Fig. 50
Ophthalmoscopic techniques: the patient's gaze should not be obstructed. A. Ask patients to fix their gaze on a distant point.
B. Inspect the fundus from above if difficulty is experienced using the non-dominant eye.

with headache, papilloedema being a feature of raised intercranial pressure. It also provides the only opportunity to visualise the patient's blood vessels. This is particularly relevant in assessing the severity of arterial changes in hypertension and the vascular complications of diabetes mellitus.

Examination sequence

❏ If appropriate, dilate the pupils using the mydriatic agent tropicamide 0.5% eye drops; alternatively, perform the examination in a darkened room.

❏ Remove both the patient's and the examiner's spectacles and make the appropriate correction for refractive errors. An astigmatic examiner may, however, need to wear spectacles.

❏ Hold the ophthalmoscope in the right hand with the forefinger on the lens adjustment wheel and use the right eye to look at the patient's right eye and vice versa for the left eye. If the examiner has difficulty using the non-dominant eye, examine the patient from above (Fig. 50B).

❏ Ask the patient to focus on a specific distant object, to breathe normally and to blink as necessary. Do not hold the eyelids open unless the patient is comatose.

❑ Keep the ophthalmoscope as close as possible to the examiner's eye with the examiner's face parallel to the patient's face. Hold the instrument as near as possible to the patient's pupil without touching the eyelashes or cornea.

❑ Keep the examiner's pupil, the aperture of the ophthalmoscope and the patient's pupil in a straight line.

❑ Rest the middle and ring fingers of the holding hand against the cheek of the patient to steady the instrument and improve visualisation of the fundus.

❑ With the ophthalmoscope lens set at zero, shine the light beam into the pupil from a distance of about 15 cm and look for the red reflex.

❑ Proceed to examine the fundus by moving the ophthalmoscope closer to the patient and adjusting the focus as necessary until the retinal vessels look sharp and clear.

❑ Locate the optic disc by following the course of an artery or a vein centrally and notice the sharpness of the edge of the optic disc, its colour and the depth of the optic cup.

❑ Inspect the arteries and veins, noting their width and colour, the light reflex along the centre of the arterioles and the appearance at arteriovenous crossings. Then follow the vessels out into the peripheral aspects of the fundus.

❑ Study the appearance of the fundus systematically by radiating from the disc to the periphery right round in a clockwise or anticlockwise manner. Note the position of haemorrhages, exudates or other abnormality.

❑ Finally, examine the macula and its surroundings by asking the patient to look directly into the light; if necessary narrow the light beam.

❑ Record the findings diagrammatically.

EXAMINATION OF A SWELLING

Masses should be examined methodically in an attempt to define the underlying anatomical and pathological features, establish a diagnosis and plan the most appropriate investigations. The mnemonic SPASECTIT may be helpful to assist examination of the most discriminant features.

- Size and shape should be recorded diagrammatically with the measurements.
- Position and its relationships to adjacent structures should be accurately defined.
- Attachments to subcutaneous and adjacent structures and its mobility or fixation should be noted.
- Surface characteristics should be defined, e.g. smooth or rough, lobulated or regular surface.
- Edge and its character should be noted, e.g. sharp or blunt, well defined or diffuse.
- Consistency is important, e.g. uniform or varied, hard, rubbery, soft or fluctuant.
- Thrills or pulsations from vascular structures or cough impulses from hernias.
- Inflammation is suggested by the presence of redness, heat, pain and tenderness.
- Transillumination of the mass with a pen torch suggests a cystic nature, e.g. hydrocele (p. 57).

NECK

The neck should be inspected for any changes in the skin, scars, swellings, and arterial and venous pulsation. The thyroid gland moves up on swallowing because the pretracheal fascia which envelops the gland is attached to the larynx. The principles involved in the examination of any swelling apply to the assessment of a swollen thyroid gland (*goitre*).

Examination sequence

❑ Sit the patient upright and examine from behind.

❑ Palpate for lymphadenopathy beneath the mandible, over the anterior and posterior triangles of the neck and above the clavicles.

❑ Pay particular attention to the scalene nodes; insert the tip of the forefinger between the two heads of the sternomastoid and feel deeply down onto the first rib (Fig. 51). Then gently pinch around the sternal component of the muscle using a finger and thumb.

❑ Palpate the thyroid gland and define the characteristics of any goitre (Fig. 52); ask the patient to swallow a sip of water to confirm that the mass moves on swallowing.

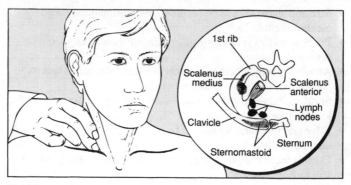

Fig. 51
Palpating the right scalene lymph nodes. (Use the left forefinger to examine the left scalene.)

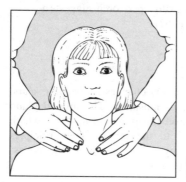

Fig. 52
Palpating the thyroid gland.

☐ Auscultate over the thyroid gland and the carotid and subclavian arteries for bruits.

☐ Complete the examination by testing neck movements (p. 105), assessing the eleventh cranial nerves (p. 94), feeling for the position of the trachea (p. 37) and inspecting the neck veins (p. 21).

BREASTS

The breasts can be conveniently examined after examination of the heart. The breast is the most common site of carcinoma in women of all age groups. Any mass should be regarded as potentially malignant.

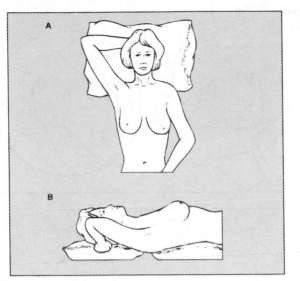

Fig. 53
Position for examination of the right breast.

Examination sequence

❏ Ask the patient to place one hand behind the head while lying flat or reclining comfortably at 45 degrees (Fig. 53).

❏ Inspect both breasts for symmetry and palpate each with the flat of the hand.

❏ Palpate the axilla carefully examining its apex and the chest wall for lymphadenopathy; use the fingers of the right hand for the left axilla, and vice versa (Fig. 54).

INTEGRATION OF THE PHYSICAL EXAMINATION

General principles

Every opportunity should be taken to learn how to examine the major systems by practising on student colleagues and on patients. Once these methods have been mastered, the student should learn to integrate them so that the patient is not unnecessarily inconvenienced. For example, while examining the limbs, the dermatological, locomotor, peripheral vascular and neurological

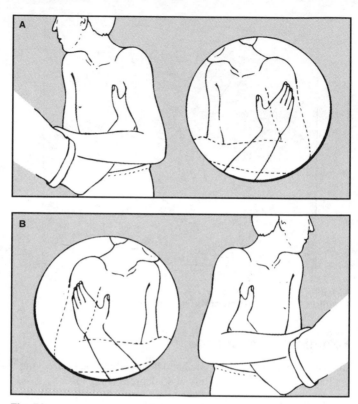

Fig. 54
Palpating axillary lymph nodes. A. Left axilla with right hand. **B.** Right axilla with left hand

components should be assessed. Any routine requires to be sufficiently flexible to be readily adjusted according to the individual problem. There is no correct sequence of performing a physical examination. Students are encouraged to modify and adapt the sequence until a method is developed which is natural. Two possible sequences are as follows:

Examination sequence – Example 1

❏ Examine the fingernails and hands, palpate the radial and brachial pulses.

❏ Examine the peripheral nervous and locomotor systems of the upper limbs.

❑ Record the blood pressure and repeat later if the blood pressure is elevated.

❑ Examine the head and neck including the eyes, ears and mouth.

❑ Examine the posterior chest including the spine.

❑ Examine the anterior chest including the heart, lungs, breasts and axillae.

❑ Examine the abdomen, groins, genitalia and perineum.

❑ Examine the lower limbs, peripheral pulses and locomotor system.

❑ Examine the joints of the lower limbs and peripheral nervous system.

❑ Examine cranial nerves.

❑ Perform ophthalmoscopy and auroscopy.

❑ Undertake a rectal and/or vaginal examination if indicated.

❑ Examine the gait and standing balance.

❑ Check the appearance of sputum and bedside chart recordings.

❑ Test the urine for the protein, glucose, ketones, bilirubin, blood and urobilinogen content.

Examination sequence – Example 2

❑ Check the appearance of sputum and bedside chart recordings.

❑ Perform an integrated examination of the lower limbs.

❑ Examine the groins and male genitalia.

❑ Examine the abdomen.

❑ Examine the posterior chest including the spine.

❑ Examine the neck and trachea.

❑ Examine the anterior chest including the heart, lungs, breasts and axillae.

❑ Perform an integrated examination of the upper limbs including the hands.

❑ Examine the head including the cranial nerves, eyes, ears and mouth.

❑ Perform ophthalmoscopy and auroscopy.

❑ Record the blood pressure and obtain blood for laboratory analysis.

❑ Examine the gait and standing balance.

❑ Undertake a rectal and/or vaginal examination if indicated.

❑ Test the urine for the protein, glucose, ketones, bilirubin, blood and urobilinogen content.

Summary points

✦ The physical examination should be adapted to suit the individual patient.
✦ There is no one correct examination sequence.
✦ Individual clinicians should use a sequence which they find effective.
✦ It is usually better to complete the examination at a later time than to exhaust the patient.
✦ Initial observations are valuable but signs are easily overlooked unless specifically looked for.

SYSTEM OF CASE RECORDING

The following provides a framework for recording an appropriate sequence of the essential findings from the clinical history and examination. Some symptoms such as breathlessness and syncope may be caused by a variety of conditions but only require to be documented once. Although the physical examination may have been 'integrated', the main findings are subdivided into the relevant systems for recording purposes and for ease of reading.

(Date and time of the examination and name of the examining clinician)

HISTORY

Personal details

Name; age; date of birth; sex; marital status; address
Occupation: patient's and, if relevant, that of the patient's partner

Past history

Previous illness episodes, investigations, therapy and transfusions
Travel abroad, immunisation schedules
Drugs and allergies
Current and recent therapy, allergies

Presenting complaint

Presenting symptoms, their duration and mode of onset

History of current illness

Chronological account of the illness up to the time of the interview

Systemic enquiry

Cardiovascular system
Breathlessness, exercise tolerance and night waking with
breathlessness
Chest pain at rest and on exertion
Palpitation, lower limb pain, ankle oedema

Respiratory system
Cough, sputum, haemoptysis
Chest pain and wheeze

Alimentary system
Nausea, anorexia and weight loss
Abdominal pain, indigestion, and heartburn
Vomiting, waterbrash and acid reflux
Odynophagia and dysphagia
Abdominal distension, belching and wind
Jaundice, stool and urine colour
Diarrhoea and rectal bleeding
Constipation and rectal mucus
Haematemesis and/or melaena

Genitourinary system
Dysuria, urethral discharge
Vaginal bleeding and discharge
Urinary urgency and incontinence
Change in urine colour and smell
Urinary frequency and nocturia

Polyuria, oliguria, haematuria
Prostatism, hesitancy, poor stream
Dyspareunia, menstrual and obstetric history

Central nervous system
Headache, visual acuity
Diplopia, hearing, tinnitus
Vertigo, dizziness, fits, faints
Paraesthesiae, numbness, weakness

Locomotor system
Joint pain and stiffness
Backache

General
Fever, night sweats, rigors
Rashes, photosensitivity, heat and cold intolerance
Excessive thirst, dry mouth, dry, red and/or gritty eyes
Sore lips and/or tongue, mouth ulcers
Raynaud's disease of the fingers and toes

Psychological
Sleep pattern, irritability
Tiredness, anxiety, depression
Memory and concentration
Libido and sexual difficulties

Personal and social history
Childhood and schooling
Previous occupations and hobbies
Housing and composition of household
Level of independence in daily activities
Support from relatives, neighbours and social services
Marriage and children
Past and current relationships
Sexual partners, number and gender
Alcohol, tobacco and/or drug use

Family history
Number and order of siblings
Inheritable disorders and family illnesses
Causes of death of family members

PHYSICAL EXAMINATION

General assessment

Demeanour and general appearance
Posture and gait
Physique and nutritional status
State of hydration and presence of oedema
Height, weight and BMI
Finger clubbing, lymphadenopathy
Thyroid and breasts
Skin and subcutaneous tissues

Cardiovascular examination

Radial pulse: rate, rhythm, volume, vessel wall, waveform
Femoral pulse: synchronous with radial, waveform
Blood pressure: supine and erect
Jugular venous pressure: height and waveform
Apex beat: site and nature
Precordial palpation: thrills, taps, heaves, impulses
Auscultation: heart sounds, added sounds and murmurs
Peripheral pulses
Arterial bruits, oedema, superficial veins

Respiratory examination

Wheeze, stridor, hoarseness, vowel phonation
Sputum: volume, purulence, blood
Chest wall deformity (pigeon chest, funnel chest and kyphosis)
Chest movement: expansion, hyperinflation (use of intercostal muscles, cricosternal distance, A–P diameter)
Trachea: displacement, indrawing and mediastinum
Supraclavicular and scalene lymph nodes
Palpation: chest expansion
Percussion: altered note and diaphragmatic movement
Auscultation: breath sounds and added sounds
Vocal resonance

Abdominal examination

Abdominal scars, pubic hair, venous distension
Distension: flatus, fetus, fat, fluid, faeces, full bladder
Abdominal movement: respiration, peristalsis
Palpation for tenderness (superficial/deep), rigidity and rebound

Palpation for liver, gall bladder, spleen, kidneys, bowel masses
Percussion: ascites, ovarian masses, bladder, spleen, liver size, shifting dullness
Examination for fluid thrill, succussion splash
Auscultation: borborygmi, bowel sounds, bruits, rubs
Hernial orifices: lymph nodes, genitalia, testicular swellings
Digital examination: rectum, prostate, vagina
Examination of stool: test for blood
Examination of the urine: test for blood, protein and glucose

Neurological examination

Mental state
Orientation, memory, general knowledge, problem-solving, serial 7s, behaviour

Speech and language
Dysarthria, sensory-motor dysphasia, dyslexia, dysgraphia, dysphonia

Cranial nerves
I   (*olfactory*):
    Anosmia
II (*optic*):
    Visual acuity; visual fields by confrontation
    Ophthalmoscopy: disc, vessels, macula
III (*oculomotor*), IV (*trochlear*), VI (*abducent*):
    Eye movements, conjugate gaze and diplopia
    Nystagmus: pendular – jerking nystagmus
                central – peripheral
    Pupillary reflexes: accommodation, light (direct and consensual)
V   (*trigeminal* – ophthalmic, maxillary and mandibular):
    Sensory: face (spinal tract segmentation)
    Motor: muscles of mastication
    Reflexes
VII (*facial*):
    Motor: muscles of expression (voluntary and involuntary)
    Taste to anterior tongue
VIII (*vestibulocochlear*):
    Hearing, Weber's test, Rinne's test
    Positional nystagmus

IX (*glossopharyngeal*):
    Sensory: taste of posterior tongue, pharynx
    Motor: salivation, gag reflex
 X (*vagus*):
    Motor: soft palate and pharynx, gag reflex
XI (*spinal accessory*):
    Motor: upper trapezius and sternomastoid muscles
XII (*hypoglossal*):
    Motor to tongue: paresis, deviation, atrophy and
    fasciculation

Motor system
Muscle power; isometric, isotonic contraction
Muscle wasting, asymmetry fasciculation
Muscle tone: hypotonia and hypertonia

Involuntary movements
Chorea, athetosis, tremors and tics

Coordination
Sensory ataxia and cerebellar ataxia
Limb ataxia and truncal ataxia, gait, rombergism
Dyspraxia

Sensory system
Spinothalamic tracts: simple touch, pain and temperature
Dorsal tracts: complex touch, vibration and position

Tendon reflexes
Supinator C5–C6; biceps C5–C6; triceps C6–C7
Abdominal T6–T12; knee L3–L4; ankle L5–S1

Supplementary tests
Meningism: neck rigidity and Kernig's sign
Straight leg flexion – sciatic nerve roots
Straight leg extension – femoral nerve roots

Locomotor examination

Posture: scoliosis, kyphosis, lordosis
Gait: osteogenic, arthrogenic, myogenic, neurogenic, psychogenic

Spine movement: flexion, extension, lateral flexion, torsion
Peripheral joints: heat, pain, tenderness, redness,
swelling–effusion
Large/small joint involvement, symmetry, active–passive
movements, crepitus
Fingers, hands, wrists, elbows, shoulders: movement, function
Hips: rotation, flexion, extension, nerve stretch tests, sacroiliac
compression
Knees: effusion, movements, collateral and cruciate ligaments
Ankles, feet and toes: flexion, extension, inversion, eversion

Clinical diagnosis

Tabulate all the relevant clinical problems.
Rank the differential diagnoses in order of probability.

Further investigations

Outline a plan of the necessary further investigations.

Sign the case notes and confirm that each page is numbered and
headed with the patient's name.

Continuing care

Record treatment plans and progress notes on a daily basis.
Record all new diagnoses established.
List any unexplained facts and the patient's active problems.
Update the problem list as the initial problems resolve and new
problems arise.
Date and sign all progress notes.

CONCLUSION

Today's 'final diagnosis' may change tomorrow because of fresh
developments or new information. Irrespective of how complete and
accurate the physical diagnosis, the individual patient may have to
make considerable readjustments in family, social or occupational
relationships as a result of illness. With some patients, physical
rehabilitation may be a lengthy process, while others may have
greater difficulty in coming to terms with the psychological impli-
cations of an illness or with the fear of its recurrence.

This book is merely an introduction to the more detailed study necessary to acquire the skills, knowledge and attitudes essential for clinical practice. For a more comprehensive analysis of the art and science of clinical examination, the reader is advised to read as widely as possible.

Recommended reading

Munro J F, Campbell I W 2000 Macleod's clinical examination, 10th edn. Churchill Livingstone, Edinburgh

Index

Trochlear (fourth cranial) nerve, 86–90, 132
Tuberculosis, 48, 116
Two-point discrimination, 82
Tympanitic percussion note, 41

Unconsciousness, 97
Upper motor neuron lesions, 70, 76, 91, 92, 97
Ureteric colic, 49
Urinary incontinence, 49
Urinary retention, 65
Urinary symptoms, 49
Urticaria, 114, 115

Vaginal bleeding, 50
Vaginal discharge, 49
Vagus (tenth cranial) nerve, 93–94, 133
Varicose veins, 15
Venous thrombosis, 15
Vertigo, 64

Vesicle, 115
Vestibulocochlear (eighth cranial) nerve, 92–93, 132
Vibration sense, 78, 79–80
Visual acuity, 84
Visual fields, 84–86
Visual impairment, 65
Vitamin B_{12} deficiency, 117
Vitiligo, 111
Vocal cord disorders, 111
Vocal cord paralysis, 32
Vocal resonance, 42, 43, 45
Vomiting, 49, 62

Weakness, 65
Weber's test, 93
Weight loss, 48
Wheeze, 33, 45
    see also Rhonchi
Whispering pectoriloquy, 42, 43
Wrist joints, 105
Xanthomatous nodules, 113